SHAPE SHIFTING

—

reclaiming YOUR perfect body

With a foreword by
Neale Donald Walsch

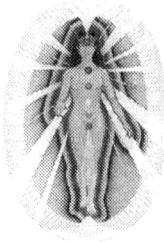

LISA BONNICE

Cover art *Aura Girl* by Justin Spyres

Shape Shifting—reclaiming YOUR perfect body
© 2007 Lisa Bonnice
1st Edition

The material inside is not intended as a substitute for a doctor or therapist. If you have health issues, or feel you could use some counseling, please do yourself the favor of getting some help.

The content of this book represents the views of the author alone. The author disclaims any liability arriving directly or indirectly from the use of this book, or any subject matter within.

Page composition/typography and cover design: Lisa Bonnice
Cover art: Justin Spyres

Bonnice, Lisa 1960
ISBN: 978-0-9799999-0-1

1. Spiritual   2. Self-help   I. Title   II. Bonnice, Lisa

Manufactured in the United States of America
10   9   8   7   6   5   4   3   2   1

Order additional copies
and get information about
the *Shape Shifters Workbook* at
www.shapeshiftingonline.com

TABLE OF CONTENTS

ACKNOWLEDGEMENTS

I finally understand what an author means when they thank people for their support. I always thought that they were just giving a shout out to friends and stuff, like saying "Hi Mom" when you're on TV. But now I know how much the support of friends and family means in an endeavor like this. Finishing this book was the hardest thing I've ever done. It's a bizarre feeling. It's a wonderful feeling. And I wouldn't have been able to experience this awesome feeling without the people who've believed in me. You all know who you are.

I do want to mention a few people by name, but I'm afraid of leaving anyone out and hurting someone's feelings simply because I wasn't thinking specifically of them when I rattled off some names. So outside of my family, I only want to mention a couple of people who specifically and directly helped me with this book. If you've been a meaningful person in my life outside of those people, you know that I wouldn't be where I am right now without you, good or bad, and I thank you for the role you've played in my life.

First, of course, I want to thank my parents for setting the stage and for being a part of my learning some of life's hardest and most powerful lessons. Being a parent is a thankless job in many ways, and I wasn't the easiest kid to deal with, but I do want them to know that I am thankful for and love them both.

I also want to thank Kristina, Stacy and Jeff (in order of appearance). I hope you've learned as much from me as I have from you.

Kristina, at one time the world's biggest skeptic, helped me to believe that I could write this book because *she* believed I could. Her own stunning Shape Shifting success is an incredible testament to what a powerful creator she is!

Stacy, my personal cheerleader and Muppet, has never doubted that I can and will do anything that I set my mind to. Her undying faith has been a god(dess)send. I hope that I have set an example to be "proud" of. (She knows why that's in "quotes.")

Jeff has been the best friend and lover that anyone could ever ask for. He is my muse. He is exquisite.

Laura Swiney has been an invaluable help. I could go on for pages why and how, but she knows what I mean. Ain't that right, Lucy?

Justin Spyres, who might as well be family, did the amazing cover art drawing of the woman and her aura. I'm honored that he took on the job because he's more talented than even he realizes. Justin, you rock!

Megan Currie, another one of my "kids," took the great photo you see on the back cover. Not only is she a gifted photographer, she's also incredible with computer art.

Outside of my family, I would like to thank Victoria Wilson for all of her guidance and teaching. Working with her has been truly life changing. I would also like to thank Beverly Combs for her help in a couple of very powerful soul retrievals, one of which directly led to the birth of this book.

Larry Trivieri, of Future Medicine Publishers, gave me the foot in the publishing door that I needed in order to learn the writing biz and James Strohecker and Burton Goldberg took a chance on me. Thanks, guys.

Ivan and Carol Dryer, inventor of the laser concert and psychic to the stars, respectively, taught me many things about being creative, daring to dream, and *never giving up*, but most of all that everyone has a story to tell.

Rick Granger and Jim Bailey at NBC33 may be surprised to see their names in here, but they gave me my start with MSNBC.com. Without Rick and Jim, I wouldn't have had such an educational and professional writing experience and therefore, the confidence that I needed to put my neck on the line.

Linda McCormick ... wow ... what can I say? Thank you, sisterfriend. I don't know if I've ever met anyone more giving, loving and filled with laughter. I only hope that I've been as good a friend to you as you have been to me. (Linda, by the way, wrote the extremely flattering text on the back cover. Another reason to value her friendship.)

Vickie Greenway (and her wonderful husband Donny), aside from being a marvelous human being, helped to pull me out of my shell and keep me out (even if she didn't realize that this is what she was doing). Not a small task! Vick, I hope we continue to talk "at least once a week" forever!

Ron Tyson and Ann Kirlan, who never got bored with the endless conversations about spirituality, kept me going during the final phases of this process. I'm so glad you two showed up in my life and I hope you stay there. El-An-Ra, indeed!

I want to thank Neale Donald Walsch, author of the best-selling *Conversations With God* series, and the man who dared to be a real life "Jerry Landers" (John Denver's character in the movie *Oh God*). I could write another entire book telling you why, but he knows. Believe me, he knows! Let's just say he embodies the word "Namaste," and I love him for it. Thank you, Neale, from the bottom of my heart and the depths of my soul.

Last, but certainly not least, I want to thank Elizabeth Anne "Betsy" Hill for her participation in a really cool, magic-filled friendship. The amazing "coincidences" that brought us together and keep cropping up have made this alliance one of the most fun times ever. Plus, without it, this publication would have been delayed even longer. Thanks, Betsy, for helping to end that agony.

Thank you one and all.

Lisa Bonnice
September 11, 2007

FOREWORD

Few experiences within the human adventure matter more to our happiness and well being than self-image. I know that it is possible for people to develop a wonderful self-image no matter what shape or size or type of body they have. Self-image has to do with our understanding of the Self that we truly are, not some exterior idea of what is "perfect" or "beautiful" or "attractive."

So the first step toward improving our self-image is to readjust the shape of our inner ideas about true beauty and wonder and even about divinity itself. You are divine, whatever shape you are in, whatever the state of your being.

Weight and shape change programs should therefore never be about "improving." It is impossible to improve on perfection—and you are perfect in the eyes of God just the way you are. They should be about changing your idea of perfection, even as you experience the perfection of your present experience. They should be about recreating yourself anew in the *next* grandest version of the greatest vision ever you held about Who You Are. In other words, while you are fine and wonderful *just the way you are,* you may choose if you wish to move to the next level in the demonstration of your personal magnificence by redefining that in any way that you wish.

What I like about the weight and shape change program offered in this book is that new tools are added to your arsenal—tools having to do with the human soul as well as the human mind and body. When we bring the soul into our life process, whatever the issue, we suddenly add a new and powerful dimension to the process itself—one that can produce utterly amazing, if not to say miraculous, results.

Spirituality IS "miraculous", and when we harness the power of God and place it into our lives in any context, we make the impossible possible. Spirituality is also fun. There is a certain joy mixed in with any expression of divinity, and that joy translates into fun and humor in the living of our day to day lives. The lighthearted approach to weight and shape change found in this book feels so good to my soul. Life is in need of a little enlightenment, it seems to me. And by enlightenment I mean the lightening up of our approach to the challenges which face us.

God is on our side. God is our best friend. When we realize this and use that power and that force in the solution of whatever our problems may be, everything changes. We no longer feel alone, we no longer feel hopeless and helpless. Here is my favorite prayer. I love it.

Thank you, God, for helping me to understand that this problem has already been solved for me.

So enjoy and embrace this spirit-centered approach to weight and shape change if weight and shape change is what you desire. I am impressed with what I see in this book. I love the nuance and the energy found here. Lisa Bonnice is a natural "enlightener." So have fun with this book, and have fun as you approach what for so many other people seems like an arduous and difficult task. Let Lisa help you make it look easy.

Neale Donald Walsch

DEDICATION

This book is dedicated to all One of us.
May it help you to remember who "we" really are.

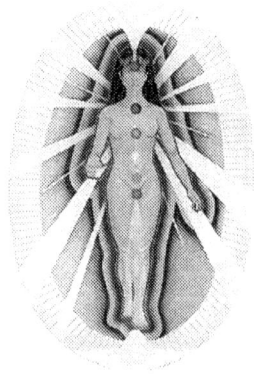

WHAT IS SHAPE SHIFTING?

Even if you're not a sci-fi fan, you've probably heard of the concept of shape shifting. For horror movie fans, it means the ability to transform yourself into an animal and back, like a werewolf or vampire bat. For those who are knowledgeable about shamanism and tribal cultures, it means working with power animals and co-joining with others for healing purposes. For fans of Star Trek or The Matrix and the like, it simply means the ability to morph into another body.

For our purposes, it means our inherent ability to constantly recreate our bodies into whatever form we choose, including our healthiest body possible—the ability to shift from a body that doesn't suit us anymore, because it's out of shape and possibly overweight, into a body that brings us great joy, using the awesome power of our thoughts. Our thoughts, which are just like magnets, bring to us exactly what we send out.

At this point in our evolution, it's not usually an instant physical transformation like in the movies, especially if we're working on something big. For now, we're still mired in the illusion of physical reality and therefore believe that we are required to follow its rules. So, we think that the only way we can change our bodies for the "better" is through horrific diets, exercise programs or—worse yet—surgery. This book is designed to help you to understand that there is another way to go about it.

The human race is beginning to wake up to the fact that there might be something to this New Age hoohah. It's not just hippies and freaks who believe this stuff anymore. There's a reason for that. It works. But until we remember how to instantly create change,[1] it takes a while for the shift to take place. So what this book is intended to do is to ease you into new thought processes that will help you to believe that you (yes, you!) can do this—that you're *already* doing it! You really can create a zingingly healthy body—the kind that feels like it's about to burst with joy, every single moment of every single day.

Having a hard time grasping the possibilities? Consider the multitude of sci-fi concepts that are now mainstream, everyday events. I believe that sci-fi is humankind's way of getting used to far out ideas, in order for the ideas to become immersed in the collective consciousness until their actualization into reality is allowed through the filter into someone's brain as an "Aha!" moment. Check out a small list of things that used to be considered stranger than fiction:

- Television and radio
- Computers
- The Internet
- Lasers
- Space travel
- Robots
- Medical body scans
- Telephones
- Walkie Talkies

[1] I believe it's entirely possible, once we learn to recognize that we're immersed in nothing but a game, with rules that can be broken.

- Holograms
- CD players

The list goes on and on. Here's something else to think about: in sci-fi, everyone is healthy or easily healed. Why is that? Could it be something else that we're eventually going to consider a no-brainer?

The most important thing to realize, before we go any further, is that shape shifting is not just a sci-fi concept. The fact is, you're already doing it! You just aren't conscious of it. Every thought, word and action causes your life to shift in one way or the other. They directly affect the shape, health and condition of your career, house, relationships—every facet of your life, *including* your body.

"Dressing for success" is a form of shape shifting. Don't be fooled by the simplicity. It really does have an affect on how you think, act and carry yourself, which then directly affects your future. Likewise, on the other end of the spectrum, living as an abused housewife will eventually affect your health, appearance, posture and extinguish the light in your eyes. Even the bestseller *The 7 Habits of Highly Effective People* follows the concepts. Deciding to change the way you think about, speak about and carry your body will specifically cause a shift in your shape.

> **At every moment, your body is in the best condition that your mindset allows.**

So you see, the idea isn't sci-fi at all. You simply need to become conscious of the fact that your body looks how it looks, and is how it is, because of thoughts, words and actions you've lived in the past.[2] At every moment, your body is in the best condition that your mindset allows. By waking up and deliberately changing your choices, instead of just going with the same flow you've been allowing so far, you

[2] No blame implied—it just is.

shift your shape to a healthier version. It also helps if you can learn to stop judging yourself and just accept that you didn't know what you were doing. You can have a fresh start any time you choose, every moment of every day.

Throughout the book, we'll be working with something I'm calling the *Essence*. You're probably familiar with the concept under various names, and I'll go into it more later, but I'd like to briefly define it up front so we are all on the same page with my specific meaning for this word. What I mean by the Essence is that substance from which our world and we are made: the liquid light—a living, breathing hologram—which flows in a never-ending, boundless river of possibility.[3]

The basic trick to making this work to your advantage is to *only* allow thoughts, words and actions that are in line with what you want to create.

If you need a visual, you might watch the move *The Matrix*—in particular the scene where Neo takes the red pill and his reality begins to dissolve into a flowing liquid. Or, watch the scenes where he dodges bullets. The ripples they leave in the air behind them demonstrate how they are moving through the substance I'm calling the Essence. When the monitors on the ship show the matrix in code, that is close to the truth of how the Essence translates our energetic impulses into what we call physical reality. While I'm aware that the storyline of this movie is fiction, it shows incredible vision on the part of the special effects department. That is what the Essence really looks like in motion. This will be explained fully, later in the book. For now, just trust me on this.

---

[3] Don't just read that sentence and not think about it. It wasn't meant to be poetic. It was a real description.

The liquidy Essence of life simply reproduces what you put into it. It responds like a giant copy machine in response to the thoughts you lay on the "glass."

Like a pebble, rock or boulder (which correspond to thoughts, words or actions) tossed into a pond, it responds with either tiny ripples in reaction to the electrical impulses of your thoughts, and/or with larger waves that your vocalizations create, and with tsunamis that your actions cause—the more active your input, the larger the result.

It's like living your life from the viewpoint of the mirror on the wall, with no judgment at all. It just reproduces what is placed in front of it. Pretend you're a mirror and pay attention to what the conditions of your life and body are reflecting through you. And know that you can change it with the flicker of a thought.

The basic trick to making this work to your advantage is to *only* allow thoughts, words and actions that are in line with what you want to create.[4] Easier said than done, right? Well, so is taking a shower easier said than done. So is reading a book, eating a meal, going to sleep…so is *everything*, no matter how easy it may be, easier said than done. But that doesn't mean you can't do it, right? We'll spend the rest of this book easing into a mindset to help you to realize that this really is easy to do, once you decide to do it.

You already know how to do this. It's just a matter of remembering to be aware of it. You picked up this book because, at some level of consciousness, you knew that there was something here for you. Trust yourself at the same level you trusted that voice inside that told you to pick up this book. (And while you're at it, give yourself a pat on the back because—congratulations—you're one of the few people who will understand this book. About nine out of ten will

---

[4] If you *fully* understand this, you can stop reading right now and begin applying that one principle. Yep, that's really all there is to it. This, by the way, is the road to Mastery.

not. The number of people who are waking up is growing, but for now it still seems to be only about 10%.)

How about an example?

Okay. I happen to have a mini example of shape shifting from real life to show what I'm talking about.

This past summer was a rough one, one that made me look and feel really old. On top of our everyday lives, with their everyday stressors, Jeff and I experienced *several* explosive events, the kinds that *individually* would have been enough to make anybody cry out to the heavens, "God, why do you hate me?" In addition, we were physically exhausted after, due to those events, living for three months in the Florida summer with no air conditioning[5] *and* moving from one house to another *twice*! I also had a job that brought me to tears on a fairly regular basis because it was so disgusting and loathsome. You wouldn't believe the details if I told you, but take my word for it: this was an exceedingly painful few months—one of the hardest periods of my entire life.

After we moved for the final time, and things seemed to have settled down, I finished unpacking and finally breathed a sigh of relief in our new, *air-conditioned*[6] place. With a fresh perspective and newly reopened eyes, I caught my reflection in the mirror and was horrified by what I saw. There were deep lines in my face that looked as though they had been etched in with a chisel and a heavy hand. I was pale and wan, and had dark circles under my eyes. My hair was dull and frizzy and I was all hunched over, like a beaten dog. In addition, my body ached all over. I was actually frightened by how much I had aged in such a brief time.

It suddenly occurred to me what had happened. I had allowed all of the "external" events and circumstances to take their toll on my physical body. Honestly, in retrospect, I don't

---

[5] Until you've lived it, you can't begin to imagine how uncomfortable a Florida summer can be without AC. It sucks the life out of you.
[6] Ibid.

think I could have prevented it because I was so deeply immersed in the hell that had become my life—I felt very distant from my soul that summer.[7] However, I realized that, in that brief period of time, I had packed years worth of living and learning into a concentrated package. I had previously, and impatiently, asked for accelerated spiritual growth and I got it![8] I may have matured 10 years mentally, emotionally and spiritually, but I didn't have to let it show physically! So I decided to see if I could erase it from my face, just for fun. No harm in trying, right?

I didn't really care if it worked. I was mostly just goofing around. I was feeling good, with all of the drama behind me, and was finally comfortable, safe and able to relax. It was more of a lighthearted effort with no real process. I simply decided to relax my muscles and let go of all the stress. I reminded myself to smile and to rejoice in the fact that all was well again. I closed my eyes and breathed in deeply, allowing the inner me to come forth.

> *You already know how to do this.* It's just a matter of remembering to be aware of it.

Much to my amazement, it worked! As I opened my eyes and watched my face in the mirror, the lines went away and my color returned to normal. The hag in the mirror was magically transformed into the youthful and energetic person that I remembered being, a long time ago (three months ago). Lest you think it was just my imagination, Jeff even noticed the difference, when he came home later. He agreed that it looked like 10 years had been removed. He had good reason for saying that—it *had* been removed!

---

[7] In fact, if you're familiar with the concept, I was going through the "dark night of the soul."

[8] Moral of the story: Be careful what you ask for.

"Big deal," you say?[9] It *was* a big deal. Remember how, when you were little, your mom told you not to make faces because your face might stick that way? She didn't realize how right she was. If I hadn't released the stress, and had continued to carry it around with me, my face would have indeed frozen that way and carried that age with it for the rest of my life—or at least until such time as I chose to release it.

This may seem like an elementary example, but it's a perfect one. The point is, this is what I'm talking about—our thoughts, worries, actions and lives in general *do* have an affect on our bodies! Maybe it's time we started to pay attention to what we're creating in every moment!

---

[9] Bravo for you if you did say, "Big deal!" That means that shape shifting will be a breeze for you and not a huge leap of faith.

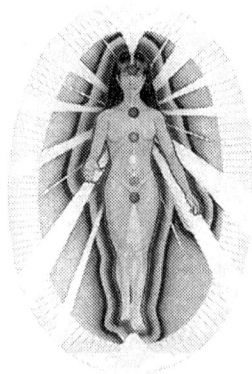

LET'S DIVE RIGHT IN!

Being unhappy with one's body, due to excess weight, is nothing more than a demonstration of a lack of understanding of one word: *love*. It really is just that simple.[10]

If we had any concept of the true meaning of the word "love" then we wouldn't be out of shape. When I say "out of shape," I don't mean needing to tone up with exercise. I mean that we are displeased and dis-eased and ill-at-ease in our body. We know that, genetically, it could look and feel a lot healthier. We have shifted into a shape that is not a representation of what we could be, at our highest point. This condition is simply a *symptom* of lack of conscious connection with Universal Intelligence, otherwise known as love—or the Essence.

The word "love" has been so misused that it no longer holds its *actual* meaning for many people. When some folks hear the word, they think of Valentines, hearts, and cupids—basically the Hallmark section of a store. Others think it means sex, heartache and/or dysfunctional relationships. Some think it means owning another person. All of these

---

[10] Stop rolling your eyes. It is, too. Read on to find out what I mean.

definitions bring relationships with others into the mix. Strictly speaking, that's not what love really is. Contrary to popular belief, love *doesn't* hurt!

If you read this book with the old definition of "love" in your noggin, you are going to totally misunderstand what I'm saying. Please don't do that. Otherwise, you might think that this is a rehashing of the old, "Fat people are only fat because they don't love themselves" routine.[11] While there is *basic* truth to that statement, it's misunderstood. It's not the romantic, hurtful love that we've been trained to think of that's the problem—it's a conscious connection to pure love energy that's missing. It's more accurate to say something like, "Fat people who are unhappy with their bodies don't love themselves." See the difference? So using the word "love" at all may be tricky. Please read this with the new definition in mind and no one will get hurt.

In fact, not all large people even *want* to lose weight, and hoorah for them, if they're happy. They may be large because they like themselves that way! But in that case, they aren't reading weight loss books, right? So, no, this book is not intended to imply that there is anything wrong with being large, or that large people all hate themselves. I hope this is enough of a disclaimer, because I would like to mush on.[12]

In a nutshell, and this will all be explained in full later, we physically feel love in the area of our body where an organ called the heart is. That is the placement of the heart chakra, which is the body's center of all of its energy flow, just as it is also the physical center of blood flow. It acts as the liaison between the upper and lower chakras (again, explained later). When this chakra is functioning and energy flows freely, then

[11] In fact, self-hatred may only come about as a result of perceived "failure" to succeed, not because of the size of one's body—which is nothing but a reminder of that failure.
[12] "Gee whiz," you ask, "What's with all the disclaimers?" Well, a book reviewer missed this point entirely when reading the first edition of the book, even though I thought I had made it quite clear. I'm making it clearer. *Capisce?*

we feel "love" energy—an explosion of happiness—a sense of expansion, where not grinning is an impossibility. As we often feel this when we're "in love" with someone, we can confuse this feeling with having someone on whom to project that feeling. Simply put, we give that someone else credit for bringing love into our life.

However, we can feel this heart centered sensation without involving other people. In fact, we're *supposed to!* We feel it when we are in touch with the Universal Intelligence—when we're soul connected. When we're in touch with that Intelligence, then we don't shift into the shape of an unhealthy body. When we're soul connected our body naturally rests at its healthiest level. Our goal here is to become soul connected *every moment* of *every day*. In order to do so, we need to find out what keeps us from it.

So when I use the word "love," I mean the energetic Essence I've spoken of already, that from which everything is made—what many call "God."[13] Therefore, for the purpose of this book, the words "love," "essence," and "god" are interchangeable to demonstrate that we don't have to struggle with the dangerously limited definitions that we've been given.

Another little replacement I've made from time to time involves the phrase "lose weight." At certain times in this book, I've used the words "gain health" instead because that's really what we're after. When we're in our healthiest form, we don't *need* to lose weight! In addition, those two little words have such a painful, negative connotation to them. I don't want to lose weight, I want to gain health!

About this book

This was originally conceptualized and written as a weight loss book—that's what I thought my "problem" was at that

---

[13] Please note the capital "G." When I spell God this way, I mean the God of religions. When I spell it with a lower case "g," then I mean the mind-blowing god source energy.

time, and it was written from that level of consciousness. So you'll see a lot of references to that process because many people still see it from that perspective.

But it became something different. It became a book about feeling good in our own skins, no matter what that looks like. So if you want to lose weight, gain weight, reshape yourself or just feel good about what you look like no matter how your body is shaped, you can use the material here—even if it may seem at times to be specifically written for weight loss. The process is the same. There are no precise diets or exercise plans, at least not for the *physical* body. Look at it as a companion guide to your dieting efforts—a metaphysical pep talk to help keep you on track.

> **When we're in touch with Universal Intelligence, then we don't shift into the shape of an unhealthy body. When we're soul connected our body naturally rests at its healthiest level.**

Therefore, you should know that the focus of the book itself is on the process that lead to my losing a significant amount of weight. It also discusses the discoveries I made about how my thoughts created a shape that I grew to hate and prevented me from shifting into a shape I could feel comfortable loving. You may or may not share the exact same process—you may wish to gain a few pounds, or just feel at peace with your current shape—and if what you read here doesn't resonate with you, that doesn't mean either of us is wrong. It simply means that those specifics aren't part of your story. The Universal Laws I followed will work for you no matter what your circumstances are, and this book will give you a clue as to how to find your story!

Like many of you, for years I dieted, starved, slaved, struggled, sweated, suffered and hated my body for not cooperating, because that's what I thought I was supposed to do. In spite of all the suffering, I *gained* weight, until I finally understood what was keeping me fat. Once I finally figured it out, I began gaining health at a rapid pace.

I didn't just wake up one day, thinner, with all this knowledge. I earned it. I learned it. I had to *live* this stuff and it works. During the writing of the first edition, I lost over 50 pounds and have continued to lose even more. I've also worked through some nightmarish health issues. I won't lie and say I did this easily,[14] like some scrawny model who says, "Mmmm, this delicious shake makes dieting yummy and look how pretty I am! It's simple (tee hee)!" I've fallen off the mountain path into the wallow pit more times than I can count. However, I gradually worked my way into allowing myself less time in the pit, so I didn't have as far to climb back out. Now I'm more on than off, where it used to be the other way around and I'm gaining health. It feels *so* good to see those numbers on the scale go down and the flabby stomach getting flatter and toned.

Sometimes we can't stick to a diet because we're too hungry or it's not going fast enough—or at all—so we say "screw it" and eat whatever we feel like, saying the next day we'll get back on. The next morning we wake up and say, "I blew it yesterday and no harm was done, so I could do it today, too, and start up again tomorrow." We can do that for months, even *years*, hating ourselves more every day because we haven't held to that resolve. We've fallen too far down the mountain to easily step back up to where we were. Now it's a major uphill battle, *again*, which we'll start climbing tomorrow.

The good news is that we don't go through difficult experiences for no reason. They are opportunities for growth. They can also be fantastic clues to whatever is in our psyches, holding us back. All we have to do is remember that we already know what it is, subconsciously, and that we can access it at any time by allowing ourselves to remember it. However, if we don't allow ourselves to remember, we keep

---

[14] I refer you back to the "easier said than done" discussion.

going through that same experience until we do. It's kind of like being held back in school. If you don't learn to read you get held back until you do. If you leave an abusive relationship, but don't change your boundaries and behavior patterns, you'll land right back into another one (and end up blaming that person's entire gender). If you go on a diet and lose weight but don't get any closer to a realization of who you really are—guess what—the weight will come right back as soon as you stop paying attention.

This is a continuing process. You don't just remember one thing and *blammo*, your body is perfect.[15] You remember one thing that helps you in one way, and then you remember the next in another way. It goes on and on. This is, I believe, the cause of those famous plateaus that dieters dread. We think we have it down to a science until the weight loss stops. After a while, we just give up because we've already cut as much out of our diet as we can bear, believing that it's about the food instead of remembering that our food choices are clues as well! But if we accept that we've grown as a result of the recent weight loss, and that we face a new fascinating challenge, we can begin again and continue our shape shifting efforts![16]

I repeat: it's not an easy road. However, it *is* easier, more fascinating and will make you far happier than the fruitless struggling you're going through now. At least I see real results to go along with the work and if I hadn't bothered, I'd still be *gaining* weight and working *even harder* to lose it, and still *hating myself.*

[15] Actually, it can be that way, but you have to have risen to an extremely high level of consciousness to realize this fully.
[16] Here's a hint. Each "lesson" brings you closer to god, because it's within our godself that the genetic memories of our healthiest selves are stored.

My story

My discovery of this process began about a year before the first edition of this book was completed. I was at my highest weight ever and at my wit's end. By that time I'd been to *countless* doctors, weight loss programs, gyms, bookstores (You should see the weight loss library I've accumulated. You too?), counted calories and carbs, used starch blockers, potato powder, and ate for my type. I bought supplements, drank diet tea, used laxatives, diuretics—pretty much everything short of bulimia and anorexia. To compound the problem, exercising literally made me ill!

This, for me, was a typical trip to the doctor:

> **Dr:** Well, what seems to be the problem?
>
> **Me:** I don't know why, but I just can't seem to lose any weight. I keep gaining and gaining, and no matter what I do, I can't lose it.
>
> **Dr:** What do you mean you can't lose it? Try dieting.
>
> **Me:** I have. I've tried every diet that looks even remotely healthy or possibly successful. I've even tried a few really strange ones with cabbage soup and hard-boiled eggs and stuff. The weird thing is, I don't even eat all that much. The people I live with eat the same amounts or more than I do and they aren't overweight.
>
> **Dr:** Everyone's different. Exercise? How often do you do that?
>
> **Me:** Not much. I just can't seem to make myself do it. I get sick when I exercise.

Dr: (Eyes rolling) What? Just do it. Instead of watching TV, you go for a walk.

Me: (knowing that's a dead end argument and changing the subject) Fine, but why can't I lose weight when I diet? Why do diets work for other people? I just get so hungry that I'm sick.

Dr: (losing patience and interest) Sick how?

Me: Nauseated, woozy, lightheaded . . .

Dr: That's your blood sugar. You should eat something.[17]

Me: Then how can I lose weight if I eat every time that happens?

Dr: (totally bored now) Here's my advice. Take these pills, join a gym and go to (insert national weight loss chain of your choice) meetings. Next! [18]

Sound familiar? I have lost count of how many times I've had that conversation with different doctors over the years - the only difference is sometimes they were downright snotty and condescending and others gave me pills that my

[17] Please note that the doctor never mentioned that these are symptoms of diabetes. I had to find that out for myself. If you have these symptoms, please ask for a test.
[18] I finally found a doctor or two who had a clue and have finally resolved some nightmare health issues that the other doctors just didn't know anything about. Moral of the story? Don't take "I don't know" for an answer. Keep looking until you find someone who does.

insurance wouldn't pay for and I sure couldn't afford![19] One actually grabbed a hunk of my abdomen and pinched it hard, saying "Look at this fat! Why don't you exercise?" as though it had never occurred to me to do so.

It doesn't help matters that some people are able to lose a great deal of weight simply through strict discipline and they have no sympathy or compassion for those who can't do it that way. They figure if they can do it, then the rest of us must be weak because their way just doesn't work for us!

No one could tell me what makes diet and/or exercise so hard to do. Why do some of us have to watch what we eat and others don't? If it's metabolism, then how come they have the lucky metabolism and we don't? *WHY CAN'T I STICK TO A DIET?*

In the meantime, I researched mind/body medicine, Reiki, holistic medicine, hypnotherapy, acupuncture, meditation, blah blah blah. I worked as an editor on a pretty well known alternative medicine encyclopedia and got to play with cutting edge technologies and knowledge. I even entered a program to get a degree in metaphysics. I gathered knowledge about how the body and mind work. Even with this focused research, I found that the amount of information available on the specific subject of holistic weight loss was miniscule.

What I did find was that we actually create illness and health with our minds. Our thoughts are just as real as the book in front of your face, and with them we create our own reality. We create our lives. We create our bodies. What we think is what we become. How we live now creates our future. There are dozens of different ways to express that same thought, and you've probably read them all if you've done any spiritual exploration of your own. And for some reason, I created an extra 75 pounds to lug around on my relatively small frame. So why did I create a fat body? And

---

[19] I find it ironic that health insurance won't pay for something that could help to make you healthier, if they have decided that it's only "cosmetic."

why can others eat whatever they want and never gain a pound?

The traditional concept of dieting doesn't apply to naturally thin people. So what's different about me? The standard answer to that is "metabolism." Their metabolism is faster than mine and burns calories and/or carbs more effectively. But why? Why them and not me? The typical response is "heredity." Okay, fine. But why then do I have an assortment of people in my family who are very thin to very large, all of whom I'm related to by blood. That still doesn't answer "why me?" So the flabbergasted response is "It's just the way you are. Deal with it."

I refuse to accept that as an answer. That dismissive response is given because *they don't know and can't admit it*. In every other aspect of life, we're expected to find our own answers. There is no reason that a weight problem should be otherwise. So I found my own answers. Throughout the rest of this book, I'll be telling more of my own story as an illustration. I hope it helps!

While this is written for both genders, there are some things that I write about that specifically apply to women. There are aspects of life that only women experience that heavily impact their body shape. Men can learn from reading about them, and comparing them to their own experiences with external influences on their bodies. Or if nothing else, they will learn a new appreciation for how hard this process is for the women in their lives.[20]

---

[20] Especially considering that men lose weight MUCH more easily than women. And we love you anyway.

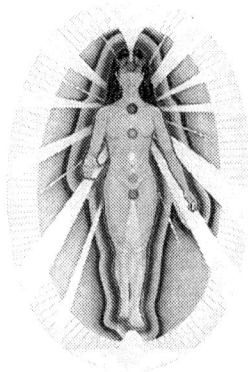

BODY IMAGE

I want you to play a little game with me. Pretend you're a blank slate. You have an androgynous, adult human body with absolutely nothing written in your memory. You know nothing about life on Earth as a gendered human being. You've been dropped into modern day society, and you have to assimilate FAST! What do you take in first?

Let's say that you hear the phrase, "You can't do anything right!" You register it as rule #1 and proceed accordingly. Then you hear the message, "Don't touch your body or show it to anyone! That's very, very bad!" which then becomes rule #2. Then you're told that your body needs to look a very specific way in order to be acceptable—rule #3.

You want to be acceptable, because that seems to be pretty important to these people you're suddenly surrounded by. But since rule #1 says that you can't do anything right, there is no way to accomplish this, or anything else, correctly. In addition, rule #2 tells you that your body is shameful, so you're not quite sure if it's okay to pay attention to what it looks like. No one else seems to be able to tell you, so you just bounce around like a pinball, trying to figure out how to follow all of the rules, especially since there are still more new rules pouring in constantly, overloading your circuits.

Tell me how you will ever achieve what you've been told is "right," if your first rule of functioning is that you *can't* do so?

With this scenario laid out for you, read on. Some of what I'm about to discuss in this section is now common knowledge, but it's only recently become so and bears repeating. Perhaps with shape shifting in mind, you'll see the information differently this time. After all, this is the garbage we've been programmed with and it's standing in the way of our healthiest form. Remember: garbage in, garbage out.

Keep in mind, also, that just because "respected" authorities say something is true, it's not necessarily so. For example, a well-known and respected 16th century Flemish biologist, named Jan Baptista van Helmont, declared that you can grow mice in a jar of wheat and dirty undies.

Describing what he called "spontaneous generation," he said, "… if you press a piece of underwear soiled with sweat together with some wheat in an open mouth jar, after about 21 days the odor changes and the ferment coming out of the underwear and penetrating through the husks of the wheat, changes the wheat into mice. But what is more remarkable is that mice of both sexes emerge (from the wheat) and these mice successfully reproduce with mice born naturally from parents… But what is even more remarkable is that the mice which came out were not small mice… but fully grown."[21]

What other "known facts" are today's equivalent? Could some of those "facts" be related to our bodies' shapes? Hmmm?

Obesity in this country is being called an epidemic and it's talked about so much that no one really even listens anymore. It's always the same thing—we eat junk and sit on our butts. Duh.

Studies have shown that in the past few decades, Americans have become heavier and heavier. It's an alarming trend that the medical world is studying; yet they haven't

---

[21] It apparently never occurred to the gentleman to put a lid on the jar to keep the mice out of his delightful concoction.

come up with any solid answers as to why this is happening. They blame fast food, lack of exercise, etc., but they don't know why changing diet and exercise doesn't work for everyone and why it has to be so damned hard!

In these same past few decades, the pressure has been *extraordinarily* strong from external sources to look a certain way, much more so than in the days before television and other mass communication media.

I believe there's a connection between the beginning of media pressure to be ultra-thin and this current "epidemic."

There have always been differing styles and body shapes in vogue, but past generations weren't inundated in their daily lives with images of gaunt models to hold themselves up to. The sheer *volume* of messages that we receive is overwhelmingly greater than ever before in our history. The energetic power of that message is more than we can metabolize. (Much more on this later . . . it's rather off topic here.)

It's easy to place blame for a poor body image on external sources, but those sources aren't the true culprits. We can point our fingers, saying they are to blame for our problems, but we *choose* whether we allow these things to affect us. It's *our responsibility* to look at our lives and not allow externals to rule us. Some of the commonly blamed entities are the media, the sex industry, the diet industry, and good old peer pressure.

Working through body image issues can seem to be an endless mass of tangled yarn, because once you uncover one bogus message that you've received and worked through, another remains buried. You have to keep digging and digging until you've removed enough of them to feel good about yourself. That's the challenge, but it doesn't have to be a drag. If you just look at yourself as a mystery to be solved, and get out your secret agent decoder ring, it can actually be a fascinating journey!

The media

It's no secret that we have all been bombarded by unrealistic images in the media of ultra-thin models. Keep in mind, too, that it's only recently that we have discovered what kind of damage has been done to the collective psyche as a result—yes, both men and women!

When I was a child, Twiggy was *the* fashion model. She was the Kate Moss of the 60's, without the heroin chic look. That's what girls were "supposed to" look like then. Imagine my dismay when I started growing hips!

> It's easy to place blame for a poor body image on external sources, but those sources aren't the true culprits. We can point our fingers, saying they are to blame for our problems, but we *choose* whether we allow these things to affect us.

My body structure just wasn't going to fit the Twiggy form and I haven't had any better luck fitting Kate Moss.' I have strong, heavy, muscular thighs. There's no getting around that. Period. Apparently I come from "peasant stock," as my dad calls it. I also have an hourglass figure—wide hips, a narrow waist, and large bust. Plus, I'm short, just over 5'2."

Now, models have surreal, massive breast implants with teeny-weeny itty-bitty little hips and waistlines. Young women and girls today have impossible-without-surgery-and/or-eating-disorder fashion images taunting them. Girls whose bodies aren't even done growing are begging for boob jobs as high-school graduation presents. Surgery has become so mainstream and common that China even holds a Miss Plastic Surgery pageant! MTV is filled with barely-dressed women, none of whom have an ounce of excess body fat or a realistic sized chest. Read any fashion blog on the net—you'll be amazed by what is called "fat" these days. Even Britney Spears is called fat by a huge number of blog commenters!

None of this is even news anymore. We all know that it's unreal and a little, but not enough, has been done to change the way things are. However, that doesn't mean that it hasn't been embedded into our psyches and those of our children.

The fashion industry

You may have had the same experience as I—attractive, affordable clothes (non-mumu's) weren't made to fit my shape until recently, so no matter what I wore, I looked fat or sloppy because clothes were always too tight in the bust and hips. If I found clothing that fit in those areas, they hung off me elsewhere.

I assumed that it must be because I'm a cow, not because clothes weren't made realistically. I can't count how many times I left the mall in tears because I was too fat, and I refused to shop in the "fat lady stores." Their clothes were ugly! Only recently have designers and stores realized that they could make money if they make clothing to fit *real* women (also known by the insulting name "plus sizes").

Ironically, I really wasn't overweight when this all started. Of course it got worse the more I gained, but I was still a size 9 when I *began* having problems finding affordable, flattering clothes. Eventually, as I kept gaining, I *had* to shop in the "fat lady stores." Oh what a horrible day it was when I first walked in the door of the plus size shop and admitted that this is where I now belonged. You want to talk about leaving the mall in tears! Well, at least I had jeans that fit.

I had an eye-opening experience at a shop once, when I could still fit into a "large." Not *one item* in the store fit me. I mean that I couldn't even get them on, not that they were a little snug. I asked the storeowner how on Earth that could be and she said that they get their stock from Asia, where the population isn't as large as Americans. All of the clothing in the store was made to fit a much smaller "large" than I was at the time. If I hadn't asked, this would have really messed with my head!

Fortunately the tides are turning, albeit very slowly. We are beginning to refuse to swallow that forced image. However, in the meantime, we still feel awful about ourselves.

The sex industry

It's not just the media and/or the fashion industry that perpetuates the impossible stereotype. The sex industry does as well. Thank you, Hugh Hefner—because you *personally* would find the vast majority of us unappealing, millions of men have been told that we're hags. And for some reason, many people (men *and* women!) have chosen to go along with that assessment.

The messages that girls and women have received for a long time is that we have to look a certain way to be sexually attractive, and boys and men have been told they have a right to demand that women look that way.[22] Both genders have been told that men only like "this" kind of woman. If I were a man, I'd be pretty doggone tired of that stereotype—they are portrayed as drooling goonboys who have no more control over their penises than a bull in full rut.

> **Thank you, Hugh Hefner—because you *personally* would find the vast majority of us unappealing, millions of men have been told that we're hags.**

So if we're "supposed" to look like Playmates in order to be sexually desirable, and very few of us do, very few of us stand a chance for a happy sex life. Sure, we might have orgasms, but we're still going to be self-conscious that our lover will notice our big thighs, fat ass, less-than-cantaloupe-sized breasts, or

---

[22] I don't want to hear about the pressure that men face to look a certain way. I have two words for you: Ron Jeremy. Do you really think that a female version would make it for one minute in the sex industry?

the roll in our gut. It's difficult to get lost in the moment when you're making sure you're lying at a flattering angle or holding your flesh in place so he won't see it jiggle.

Good news though—I've found from experience and through asking around that men (not boys—I specifically mean *mature*[23] males) are usually perfectly content with their women, and a good lover really doesn't bother to look for fat when their minds are on what they're doing. Many only notice what we consider to be excess weight because we insist on constantly pointing it out to them!

On the flip side, if you have a mate who belittles your body, then *that* person has the problem. Making fun of another is cruel and immature, even if they say, "I'm doing it to motivate you." And if they do say it's motivation, then it's your right *and* responsibility to tell them that it hurts and motivation doesn't work that way. Usually, it just drives us back to the stash of food we've hidden.

We should also remember that we simply cannot compare ourselves to media images because those women are *unusual*. Look around you. How many women do you see in real life who look like that? Very few—even *average* sized women don't look like that. And they're called average for a reason. They're **average**! The **average** woman is a size 14 and the average **model** is in the low single digits. We're shooting for an extreme—one that a small number of people will *ever* reach!

Yet we continually compare ourselves to the dancers on MTV and bony model types, and on and on.

Bodies like theirs don't commonly occur in everyday life. These women are dancers and models. It's what they *do*. They devote their lives to looking like that. They may have personal

---

[23] And I don't mean "old." I mean mature—someone who has evolved past the drooling goonboy stage. I know a lot of old farts who still qualify as "goonboy."

trainers, possibly eating disorders,[24] and their daily job is to sculpt and move their bodies. Their very livelihood depends on their looking like that. Many of us sit at a desk and actually *eat* once in a while. It's **insane** to think you'll look like them without following the same strict "discipline."

Nudity

Many women can't even stand to look at themselves in the mirror naked. They're repulsed by what they see.

One of the most eye-opening things I've ever done is to become a nudist. Jeff and I went to a nude beach for the first time in the early 90's. I was worried sick. At that time I was only about 20 pounds over what I wanted to weigh and I thought I'd be the biggest heifer on the beach. I worried about people laughing at me, or sneering and wondering, "What does she think she's doing here?" I also worried that he was going to be surrounded by all these dazzling beach creatures, totally nekkid, and was going to suddenly find me absolutely repulsive. This was even after he spent *hours* reassuring me that this wouldn't happen.

I was delighted to find, when we got to the beach, that nobody there had the body I expected. There were all different shapes, sizes, colors, ages, scars, etc., and everyone was totally relaxed. One woman even had one breast that was smaller than the other. I loved that she was as comfortable there as anyone else.

There was no sexual tension, because nudism isn't about sex. It's about feeling good in your own skin—being real. There was no self-conscious tugging of too-tight suits, or hiding fat body parts. In fact, there was one woman who was built like the Venus of Willendorf—massive thighs, good sized gut, huge breasts. She was tanned and her hair was sun-bleached. She was chasing her little, tanned tow-headed kids

---

[24] I don't want to imply that all slender women have eating disorders, but we're talking about the media, and let's not kid ourselves for the sake of being politically correct.

around on the beach, playing Frisbee. She was beautiful—completely at ease with her woman's body. She had stretch marks and all the obvious signs that she'd had a couple kids. She was *real*. And she was *happy*.

The diet industry

There is a gazillion dollar diet industry telling you that you're too fat. There are boatloads of cash to be made off of your insecurity. If you drink this, or eat that, or swallow this, or pay for that, you'll be thin and beautiful and therefore a better person. Children and puppies will love you more, and your lover will stop the roving eye. Life will be good and the angels will sing.

The problem that I see with some diet plans is that they promote fantastic instant gratification. Betty lost 40 pounds in two weeks! Jeanette lost 120 pounds in eleven days! Huge promises with very little wait time.

Of course, there is the obligatory microscopic print, "*Results not typical,*" which flashes by very quickly. No kidding, the results aren't typical! If they were typical, no one would be overweight and the companies who promote these plans would win some sort of Nobel Prize for curing this problem. If diet potions and concoctions worked

> **There are boatloads of cash to be made off of your insecurity.**

that well, we would have heard about them from people other than the company promoting that program. The inventor of such a plan would be wealthier than Bill Gates.[25]

I saw a newspaper ad for one of the major weight loss chains where they pictured a woman in a leotard, looking very slender. However, when I looked closely at the ad, I saw that they had taken her real outline and faded it out, so the printed dots were further apart and at first glance she looked thinner than she really was. In addition to being dishonest, this ad

---

[25] Who is, by the way, $7.84 short of being wealthier than God.

was belittling the hard work that she had accomplished, as though she *still* wasn't thin enough, when the shape she actually had was just fine!

The "before and after" pictures bother me too. The before pictures usually show someone fat and frumpy, wearing sloppy clothes and no makeup, hair like a fright wig. She's usually stuffing food into her face. The after pictures show her in a bikini with her gut sucked in, her hair all poofed and coiffed and makeup flawless. In essence, they're showing us that we're worthless and ugly before we use their product.

A woman in a man's world

Guys, you can skip this part if you want, or you can read on to find out what the women in your life go through. This may not seem to have anything to do with weight, but it really does. It's a body *shape* issue. I should add, also, that this is coming from the perspective of someone born in the 60's. Much of this has changed for younger women, thankfully, but they still have their own versions of sexism to deal with.

For me, being a girl meant being treated like a second-class citizen. It meant having to clean the house instead of being able to build something out of wood, or having to wear a shirt on a really hot day, even with puberty years away. In fact, when I was in non-parochial elementary school, girls were still required to wear dresses or skirts. The only time we were allowed to wear pants was if we had gym class in the morning, but we had to change back into a dress at lunch time.

I wanted to climb trees and do the fun stuff the boys got to do. I was also belittled if I did do "girl" things, or if I threw "like a girl." Basically, being a girl wasn't a good thing. Your primary purpose in life was to cook for and clean up after the men, and to look good doing it (with your mouth shut, of course). There didn't seem to be any way to win.

Our fathers bought into this, making things even worse. The man who teaches you how a woman should be treated— the man who is supposed to love you more than any other—

is telling you that you're not as good as the boys. Our mothers lived this way with him, apparently agreeing. Therefore, you're also getting that message from your female role model. Who can fight that? What choice, as a kid, did you have?[26] But that's how the world was back then. It's our responsibility now as adults to acknowledge that this is the way it *was*—that we have it within our own power to live differently and to teach our children otherwise.

Problem is, kids these days are getting an entirely different, yet equally as harmful message. Now, girls are taught that being slutty is the way to display their empowerment. Don't get me wrong. I'm not necessarily talking about revealing clothing. I'm talking more about the attitude. I'm all for empowerment, and am happy that female sexuality/sensuality is finally beginning to awaken again. However, I think they're missing the mark—they're trying to do it through the male perspective—they're practicing what they believe men want, instead of as a true expression of their womanhood. They think they can demonstrate these things just by wearing lots of makeup, tight-fitting and skimpy clothing, and having random sex. No one is telling them that the difference between slutty and sexual/sensual is a love of self. They're doing it to *impress* boys, not to *express* the Goddess within. Big difference—*huge* difference!

As a result, many girls and women gain weight to hide their femininity, which implies either being nothing but a second class citizen, or a sex toy. It's okay to be considered attractive, or to have someone look at you admiringly, or even with sex in mind. But if you're insecure, you feel dirty when you're *leered* at, as though the person leering assumes that you would pretty much have to do whatever they wanted and it would be all for *their* pleasure, almost a visual rape.

---

[26] Let's not blame our parents though, because they were only living what they were taught—just like we are. We pass on our revised versions of this garbage to our own kids.

Is it any wonder some of us gain weight, so they won't look at us like that? It's a twisted power statement, as if we're saying "I may not be able to protect myself from you, but I can make you stop wanting me that way."[27] The subconscious does screwy things sometimes, things that don't make sense to the logical mind. Rape or incest victims commonly gain weight as their way of making themselves less attractive to men. Some go the opposite direction toward anorexia and starve themselves so they won't look sexual at all. In fact, they even stop having their periods and their bodies lose any signs of being a mature female.

Age

Unless we die young, we get old.

Did you just respond with a hearty, "Duh!"? Well, if it's so obvious, then why are you killing yourself to look young? Why is there such a fear of aging? Unless you die early, you're going to get older! Your body will only look 17 when you're near that age. You will not look 17 when you're 30. Accept it. Go ahead and remain youthful and vital, but don't become so obsessed that you hate yourself because your breasts sag a little. It's what breasts do in a gravitational environment. Remember, Hollywood is not reality.

How does all this affect us?

All of these things silently and gradually chip away at your self-esteem and personal strength. If you only feel physically valuable if you look a certain way, but you don't feel strong enough or worthy of looking that way, then you'll *never* shift into that shape because you feel you don't deserve to. Or if you feel *vulnerable* looking that certain way, you'll do whatever it takes to look otherwise, even sabotage your body by

---

[27] I do not mean to imply that only "sexy" women are raped. We've all heard horror stories of senior citizens, children, nuns, women of all shapes and sizes, and even boys and men, being raped.

shifting into a shape that you hate. But at least you feel safe. Whew! What a mind twist!

We hang on to these lies because if we strip away all of the reasons that we don't feel good about ourselves, we have to replace them with something. We're left exposed and empty unless we replace these things with new information. If we don't know what to replace them with, we don't remove them in the first place. This book will help you to replace them.

Remember that just because one person says something is true for you, it's not necessarily so. Einstein failed math as a child. But perhaps it was just too basic for him. Maybe when the teacher said, "Two plus two equals four," little Al was thinking, "Not necessarily." What typical teacher wouldn't mark that response as incorrect?

Keep an open mind as you read. And prepare to have it blown.

False media image

We must remember that the body we have is our own, and it's not *ever* going to look like any other. Period. Just like snowflakes and fingerprints are all unique, so is our DNA and, therefore, so are our bodies. It's a simple fact and there's not a thing we can do about it. Even identical twins have differences.

Once we can accept that, we realize that there's not a thing we should *want* to do about looking "better" for a group of strangers. My body is as good as any other, even if it's "over weight," and so is yours. Why we should allow some temporary societal pressure to cause us to hate our bodies is beyond me. And it *is* temporary. Marilyn Monroe was a size 14. During the 1600's, Peter Paul Rubens painted plump women, who were considered to be attractive at that size (this is where the phrase Rubenesque originated). Being heavy, then, was a sign of beauty because it meant that you had wealth and, therefore, food.

Some concepts of beauty were downright dangerous! In the "old days" women wanted to look like they had tuberculosis, foot binding was considered sexy and corsets were everyday wear!

Tuberculosis—also known as consumption—was common among artistic people and it became fashionable. Lord Byron even wrote, "I should like to die of consumption. The ladies would all say, 'Look at that poor Byron, how interesting he looks in dying!'" In the mid 1800's people thought getting TB meant you were spiritual and refined. As you became weaker and wasted away, the theory goes, your spirituality was revealed.

Tuberculosis caused a pallor, which indicated wealth because tanned skin meant you were a poor field-worker. However, once life became industrialized and workers came inside, they became pale and the wealthy got tans, because only they could afford to take time off and lie in the sun.

Foot binding occurred in China for centuries. The most common explanation that I've found is that a dancer for the emperor bound her feet in silk, creating a fashion. She was known for her beautiful tiny feet too, so the binding and the size became the focus of the fashion. The sizes were forced smaller and smaller as time went on. Eventually girls' feet were bound tightly with cloth strips to keep their feet from growing any larger than four inches. The four smaller toes were broken and the foot was folded in on itself to keep it shortened, thereby crippling the girl.

Only the wealthy could afford to not be able to walk and many poor women, who needed their feet to survive, would have their feet bound in order to be considered suitable for marriage. Unfortunately, many of them remained poor and still had to work with their crippled feet.

Tiny feet were considered beautiful and even erotic. There are tales of men drinking the footbath water and it was a believed that a woman who walked with bound feet would produce a strongly muscled vagina. Sexual guides included techniques to use the bound foot for sex.

Corsets, a common item of women's clothing at one time, caused the ribcage to overlap and the internal organs to be compressed. Women strove for a "wasp waist" and tightened their corsets beyond a reasonable, healthy amount, in the name of fashion. They crushed the lungs and made it difficult to breathe properly, which goes a long way toward explaining why women "swooned."

Think about these examples and then consider what forms of torture and starvation you've put yourself through. In a hundred years from now, hopefully sooner, people will be just as shocked at what we do, as we are to hear of these old fashions. "They did what? What were they thinking?"

I want to be as fit and healthy as *my* body is able and that is *my* personal best. No one has the right to ask for more than that from me, *including me!* I will never look like a model unless I starve myself, get lots of surgery and spend a week being stretched on the rack. Personally, I don't think it's worth it.

The mistaken sex industry

The next step is facing the mainstream sex industry's image of women. Somehow, they've decided that the previously discussed body style is the only sexy one and huge numbers of women have gone along with it. This is the way it is, *for now*. But until it changes, are we going to believe that we aren't sexy because we don't look like airbrushed centerfolds and—even at our personal best—we never will? This thought pattern implies that we're not good enough to enjoy sex, or even HAVE sex for that matter, unless we look like their twisted ideals.

Ask some of the men you know. You may be amazed at how they really don't expect us to look like that. Many men are even sexually attracted to what they call "Big, beautiful women" (BBW). If you watch X-rated movies, try renting the "amateur" ones with real people, not porn stars. You might even surprise yourself with your initial reaction of, "Who wants to watch fat people have sex?" especially if they really aren't *fat*. You might even find it disgusting. That's your own knee-jerk reaction in an effort to conform to that societal stereotype, projecting your self-loathing onto them. But what you'll find, if you give it a chance, is that these people are really enjoying themselves and aren't worried *at all* that they don't look "right." Don't you want to be able to do that?

The best part is that, once you get past these issues, sex is a whole new ball game! You can't begin to imagine how much better it is when you're not freaking out over your appearance! You don't have to be beautiful to have killer orgasms, even though many people think so. Appearance has absolutely *nothing* to do with your ability to enjoy sex except in your own head.

> **Are we going to believe that we aren't sexy because we don't look like airbrushed centerfolds and—even at our personal best—we never will?**

Orgasm is humankind's method of communicating with Universal Intelligence—it's not just for relieving horniness. Why do you think we say, "Oh, god!" during sex? The more open you are to that Intelligence (that openness requires that you love yourself—see yourself as the Essence you are), the more powerful orgasm is.

In addition, the concept of sex magic becomes a reality. You do not want to even attempt it if you don't feel good about your body. More on that later!

Sexism and fat

Being in a female body is something that you can't do anything about (sex change only changes your appearance), so if you're angry at being a woman, at being discriminated against or being treated as a sex object, then you're going to have to work on personal strength—being able to feel like you can stand up straight and take on the world.

I bet everyone with the "ideal body" has had this experience at least once, that of not being taken seriously because the person they're talking to is too busy trying to put the moves on them. Women in particular know what this is like, especially if you're dressed attractively. Many men will not hear you, and will just think of you as a fluff chick or a future conquest. However, look how much they pay attention to what big women say—there's not usually a lot of sexual energy or tension there, so the woman has a better chance of being heard. Many bigger women are thought of as being bossy. I think it's because we subconsciously assume that gaining weight is the best way to get people to listen to us so we shift into that shape. Perhaps the bossiness comes as a result of subconscious anger at being "forced" to be fat, just to be heard.

Here's another aspect of the issue. Look at the comedienne Roseanne. She's large, so she's called a bitch. Other performers with "sexier" bodies are called divas for the *exact same behavior.* While diva isn't necessarily a label I'm shooting for, I'd much prefer it to bitch. A bitch is reviled. A diva is feared. If I had to choose between the two, I'd rather be feared because at least there's an aspect of respect involved. However, given my druthers, I'd be in a healthy body and respected because I respect myself and thereby command the respect of others.

I spent seven years touring as a standup comic. In my experience, there was a general preconceived notion in the industry that women aren't as funny as men. Women comics weren't as desired by clubs and it was a rarity to have more than one woman on the bill unless it was advertised as "Ladies Night." I recall a club owner of a famous Chicago comedy club saying "(Women)[28] ain't funny." But if you're pretty and have a nice body, it's even worse. The crowds and club owners don't expect you to be funny so you don't get work. Heavier women don't have that problem to the same

---

[28] He didn't actually use the word "women." He used the dreaded "C" word.

degree, so it's easier to get work and audience respect if you're fat. Isn't that odd?

If you've had similar experiences of not being taken seriously because of attractiveness, you may have even gained weight as a form of revenge. You're showing them, "Look what I've become, because you hurt me. I'm fat because you made me feel bad about myself." Another form of this revenge against the Playboy image could be, "I don't have to look like that mold you're forcing me into. I'll be fat if I damned well please, and you can't do anything about it."[29]

This is a form of control. If you feel that you have little control in your life, and your weight is one of the few things you can control, here come the pounds. The same is true in many cases of anorexia—girls will starve because it's the only part of their lives that they feel they *can* control.

The problem with that kind of control, though, is that it's harmful. In the end, we really can't control anything in life as long as there is at least one other person involved. Total control is only something you can have over yourself, and even then it's tricky. Only you control your actions and reactions, your thoughts and feelings. Allowing others to belittle you into gaining weight is actually a sign of NOT being in control. You're letting *them* control your reactions.

Bottom line

What this all boils down to is that, sometimes even if you already have your "perfect body," you've been told by practically *everyone* that you're fat and that your body isn't good enough. Later we'll get into how these thoughts have power. We've *literally thought ourselves fat*. Ask and ye shall receive. But be careful what you ask for!

---

[29] That was one of my big issues. I was so mad that I was "expected" to look like *that*, that I proved that they couldn't make me. However, "*they*" are a fantasy. They're a figment of my imagination, because there really isn't a panel of people sitting around deciding what Lisa should look like.

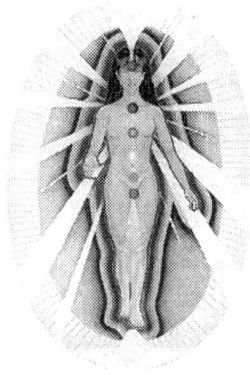

THE PHYSICAL BODY

Physical problems that shouldn't be ignored

This book is about the *metaphysical*[30] causes of weight gain
and loss, not on cures of diseases or treatment of *physical*
causes of weight gain. You won't find charts, graphs, stats or
discussions about cholesterol or blood pressure, etc.

However, physical conditions, including hormonal
imbalances, thyroid problems, diabetes, heart problems,
morbid obesity, etc. shouldn't be ignored. We will discuss the
metaphysical causes of illness later, but please don't wait until
you fully understand how it works in order to see a doctor
and get any treatment that might save your life.

While you're working with your doctor to keep any health
conditions under control, we'll look at what may be some
underlying causes.

No diet plan here!

Let's get this out of the way first. If you're hoping to see a
diet laid out for you, like "have a half a grapefruit (no sugar)
with dry whole-grain toast and skim milk," throw this book
right out the window (after you throw out that god awful

---

[30] Metaphysics means "beyond the physical."

37

breakfast). You're not going to find any specific diet graphed out for you here. You must decide, by listening to your own body and taking responsibility for it, what you eat.

I'm not going to pretend to know what's best for you, or that I'm a nutrition or exercise expert. Chances are good that you've already read up on the subject until your eyes are swimming in your head. You could probably earn a degree with all the information you've gathered. I can recite the food pyramid in my sleep and I know what foods give me certain reactions, both good and bad. In fact, Elson Haas, M.D., has written that, many times, food reactions can be the culprits that make us gain weight. I recommend his book *The False Fat Diet* for more information.

I, personally, found his "diet" to be very helpful for me. Through the process of elimination, I was able to find out what foods will trigger eating binges, bloating, stuffy nose, fatigue, etc. I was amazed at how much better I felt and was able to stay with this way of eating because I felt so good AND was gaining health.

That does not mean that it wasn't hard in other ways. I still had my issues to overcome, and my battles to wage. I still felt like pigging out when I was mad, sad, depressed, angry, happy, etc., but it wasn't out of hunger. Also, I was able to easily slide back into this way of eating after a binge—it only lasted for a day or so, no longer. I remember binges that lasted six months!

Here's the short version: Do your research. Eat what you know is healthy for *you*, in portions that you know are healthy for *you*. Simple as that. You're a grown up.[31] You can make this decision for yourself, without some diet guru telling you what you must or must not eat. Be willing to learn by trial and error what works and what doesn't. *No one knows better than you what is healthiest for your body.* Peer pressure is pretty powerful (what a lot of alliteration!), and our friends and family may

[31] This actually comes as a surprise to some people—they live their lives feeling like a child with no power.

really push us to eat what they're eating. Giving in is your choice. You are the one who pays the consequences, not them. It's *your* shape that you're shifting with your choices, not theirs.

Exercise

Regarding exercise (chorus of hisses and boos), I'm not going to tell you to go pump some iron. If you want to become muscular and finely toned, then I honestly don't know of a better method.[32] But if you just want to look healthy, there are many other things you can try. Maybe you just want to be in shape, to not have your thighs and gut jiggle. In order to find the right form of exercise, you need to do some soul searching.

> **Movement is literally our muscles' way of expressing themselves. It is what they do, who they are—their *raison d'être*. The tone and strength of our muscles are the physical manifestation of how we care for our bodies**

I bet you're stiff and sore all the time. The idea of exercise isn't appealing because it hurts and is extremely uncomfortable. The goal of exercise seems to be to make yourself uncomfortable for as long as you can bear it. The payoff is that you will be able to go for even longer stretches of time being uncomfortable. Woohoo! Sign me up!

Your body is stiff and sore because you haven't moved it or used it in a very long time. The longer it's been, the more it hurts. But can you remember a time when you were limber? Even if you were a heavy kid, you tried to do cartwheels or move somehow until you got so heavy that you just couldn't anymore.

---

[32] That doesn't mean one doesn't exist.

Movement is literally our muscles' way of expressing themselves. It is what they do, who they are—their *raison d'être*.[33] The tone and strength of our muscles are the physical manifestation of how we care for our bodies—how we allow them to be what they are. If we don't care for our muscles, they will be weak and flabby. They will shift "out of shape."

If we have the use of our muscles, instead of having lost them through accident or illness, then we should appreciate them and let them do what they love to do. Our muscles love to move and it can feel really, really good. Let them!

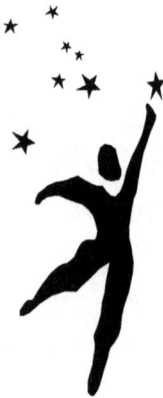

Many diet books will give you a list of things you can do other than weight lifting, like going for walks, roller-blading with the kids, climbing stairs instead of using the elevator, or parking as far from your destination as you can. Beautiful, if that's what you like to do—I'd rather eat worms. However, when I was younger I loved to dance.

As a teen I took dancing classes and performed in dance revues. As an adult, I had a job as a waitress in a place where once an hour we did dance routines to songs from the 50's. After work, we'd all go to a nightclub and dance 'til we dropped. Dancing has always been my favorite form of exercise, because I didn't consider it to *be* exercise. It was simply the way I most enjoyed moving my body. However, my life has changed and that's not a possibility anymore. Now I am satisfied with belly dancing classes and I do go to the gym, even though it's a battle to go because I find it extremely dull. I find, however, that if I visualize my body getting healthier and my muscle groups getting stronger as I work out, it becomes a form of prayer, or meditation.

[33] Hey, look! *Je parle français!*

40

If you haven't exercised in a long while, yoga is a great way to wake up the body into being alive and mobile again. Even gentle stretching, T'ai Chi or Qi Gong (also spelled Chi Kung and other variations) are fine ways to move your muscles. They are energy exercises and are perfect for easing into exercise. Your muscles need to be awakened after their long slumber.

Really *feeling* your muscles moving and *imagining* them strengthening in your mind's eye is immensely helpful. If you gently ease your body into movement, you may gradually be able to work your way into something a little more strenuous. Your muscles will *absolutely* respond to this new care you're giving them. They *will* shift into shape. They can't help it—it's Universal Law.

Ease into it. Think about how you feel when someone jars you awake—sometimes you get angry, other times you're startled—however you react, it's not pleasant. But if someone gently wakes you, maybe gives you a kiss on the forehead, or some other sign of affection, then you're not going to mind waking up so much. You can think of your muscles the same way. If they are suddenly jolted into a half hour on the exercise bike they'll rebel in a like manner. They'll get stiff and sore and you won't exercise again.

You don't have to be like Suzanne Somers with her Thigh-Master right away. In fact, you *can't* be like her right away! Do what you love, what your body loves. Find your joy and bliss again in moving your body. Do what you loved to do as a kid, and if you need to work into it slowly, love yourself enough to give yourself time to do so. You may not believe this, but I finally worked up to a point where I really love doing crunches. It feels so great to be able to do it and really control the muscles. I found that really good stretches in the crunch position make my lower back much stronger too and that's an area where I had serious trouble. (Don't take this as medical advice. If you screw up your back doing crunches, it's not because I told you to do them, it's because you chose to do them incorrectly.)

There's plenty of time later to knock yourself out at the gym, if that's what you choose to do. But if you start out that way, it's going to hurt and you're going to hate it and then you're not going to do it. You will get better results if you lovingly awaken your body first.

Here's something I was stuck on and only recently figured out: I lived in my head. I was much more interested in thinking and reading and "pondering deep thoughts," than I was in being physical. I'm not a real fan of sports, I don't like competition, I'm not interested in skiing or other forms of exercise where you can get hurt, and I don't like being sweaty. I valued meditation and energy work and all the really amazing, cool things you can do with your brain when you work to develop your psychic skills. I only worked on honing that craft and am now pretty good at it. However, my body suffered.

We need to be physical just as much as we are mental and emotional. It's the "holy trinity" and if you leave the physical out, then the body makes up for it by weighing you down. It's literally *forcing* you to stay grounded. This is why it's not necessary to kill yourself with exercise to make progress. Just be physical! We're the opposite of the stereotypical "dumb jock," who is mostly physical and doesn't use the mental abilities he/she has. So if you look at people who have great bodies as stupid, this may be why. You're projecting your fear—that of being perceived as having a nice form and no brains—onto them.

Even deeper (every issue is multifaceted), my refusal to be physical was part of my rebelling against being forced to be the only kid to clean the house because I was the only girl and housework was "women's work." If the house needed to be cleaned, as an adult, I'd go sit down and write instead, or do something else "important" . . . more important than such a menial task as cleaning. Someone else could do it, or I'd get around to it when I was done with my "important business" (which was never finished, by the way). I made money with my brain, and didn't get paid to clean the house. So being physical in this way, moving and exercising in this way, was demeaning to me.

I valued my thinking much more than my physical world because that's what the boys got to do. They were encouraged to go to school and be something, I was encouraged to keep a nice house and *find* someone who went to school and did something. I *hated* cleaning the house for that reason. By extension, I hated that form of exercise. So even my messy house was a symptom of why I couldn't gain health!

The whole point of this section is *just get up and move.* Some how, some way—it doesn't matter. Just move your body. While you're doing it, appreciate the progress you're making! Once you start to actually see a difference (if you've got a long way to go it's very subtle at first) rejoice in the change! Look at what you've done and give yourself a pat on the back. Don't look at yourself in comparison to how you *want* to look down the road. Look at how you *used to* look, before you started. Once you start to see the tiniest bit of definition, you'll want to see more and you'll *want* to exercise. You'll find that walking feels good, because you can feel your muscles propelling you forward. Lifting things will be a pleasure because you have the strength to do so. Enjoy the shape shifting progress instead of bemoaning how far you have to go. You'll get there eventually, but for now you deserve a lot of credit for making the effort. Baby steps.

> ## Don't look at yourself in comparison to how you *want* to look down the road. Look at how you *used to* look, before you started.

Eating with the family

I got lucky in that Jeff loves to cook.[34] However, he also loves to eat fattening, starchy foods. He's a meat and taters

---

[34] I'd rather just open a package of something.

kind of guy. So unless I want to cook my own separate meals, I eat what he makes. These meals usually consist of some sort of meat, potatoes or pasta, gravy, usually corn and biscuits or rolls and lots of butter—a *major* starch and carb fest. All the foods are brown, white or yellow. And he *hates* the kind of food I love, which falls under the general heading of "health food." He calls it "bean curds and dirt."

He *piles* food on the plates. Mountains of food that would feed a small army would appear in front of me. In spite of my many protests, he would keep scooping it on. I used to tease him that he wants me fat, and maybe somewhere deep inside he does, but in the end it's me who finishes all that food or not. It's up to me to say "when." Would it hurt his feelings if I don't eat all that he gives me? At the risk of sounding cold, that's not my issue. Will it hurt my body if I do eat it all? *That* is where it becomes my problem.

However, the majority of households still have the woman doing all the cooking, and usually she's preparing what the family likes and wants, not what she personally needs and wants to eat in order to make her own cells sing. She sacrifices what her body tells her in order to keep the peace in the household.

In all of the weight-loss programs that I've joined, the group meeting includes at least one person saying that the family doesn't like her "diet food." It's therefore hard to stay on her diet as a result. She is not serving herself, but is instead serving her family's desires. Ironically, what they're asking for may not be what their bodies need, but instead what their *mouths* enjoy eating. Happily, there are many good replacements for the old foods, and most of them will pass without the family even knowing. Drop by your local health food store to see what you can find.

We need to learn to take care of ourselves. If we don't, no one will. Jeff would be happy to make what I like and want in addition to his food, but I don't feel like I should ask him to do the extra work, because he's already making a meal. I don't ask him to make my favorites *instead* of his, because he can't stand them, and my *mouth* likes what he makes (even though it's not what's best for me). For a long time, I also couldn't rationalize spending the money on the extra food it would take to keep me feeling my best. I wasn't serving myself. And it was no one's fault but my own.

In order to change the foods you eat, *you must take charge.* For the longest time I was afraid to spend the money on the food I really wanted. I was afraid he would get mad at me. (This is a throwback from my first marriage where my ex would get mad if I spent money on paper towels!) It took more than 10 years for me to realize that he didn't get mad when I bought healthy food. So I started doing so and it makes eating healthy *so* much easier, just having the food in the house, instead of skulking out to the health food store once in a while and sneaking what I needed.

This was a pretty deep issue for me. I finally realized that I was projecting my feeling that my needs weren't important onto him. He never, not one time, said that I couldn't buy what I needed. It was all my fear of rejection that kept me from even bringing it up. However, if you are involved with someone who will get angry, or your budget is such that you simply cannot afford to buy "health food," then this goes much deeper. Weight gain can be a subconscious statement of, "Okay, fine. You won't let me buy the foods I need, so I'm going to get fatter. See how you like them apples!" Personally, I like them apples dipped in caramel.

Lack of money, though, is another massive, painful issue that many people struggle with. Sometimes it's harder to deal with than being overweight. Haven't you seen people who are obviously financially poor but are dangerously obese? Have you wondered how they can afford to eat enough to get so big? I've even heard people in grocery store lines talking about folks in front of them using food stamps, saying that if they didn't eat so much and spend so much on food, they wouldn't be poor. But it's not always from overeating. Many times it's from the poor nutrition that comes with cheap food. That poor nutrition is what causes food reactions and cravings, thereby causing weight gain. They just don't know how to shop and/or eat right.

If, instead of spending your hard-earned money on junk food and gut stuffers, you bought the kinds of foods that keep you healthy, then the cost wouldn't be much different. In addition, by eating the right foods for you, the cravings go away and you don't have to wage the battle of denying those cravings, which make gaining health next to impossible.

In order to serve ourselves, we need to ask why it's so hard to buy and prepare the foods that *we* need to be healthy. I've just discussed the buying, but I had to also figure out why I hate to cook and clean. If I had a personal cook—someone dedicated to shopping for, preparing, and cleaning up after healthy meals that fit within my guidelines, seven days a week, without my having to lift a finger—I wouldn't have a weight problem. Neither would most of us. So this tells me that it goes deeper than just the foods I eat. It's the foods I *choose* and the lack of care that I take of myself. Why can't I be that personal cook?

> **In order to serve ourselves, we need to ask why it's so hard to buy and prepare the foods that *we* need to be healthy.**

That's an easy one, actually. Going back to the way I was raised, the woman does *all* the cooking. The man sits at the table and waits to be served, which always made me furious. Apparently it was a strong enough issue for me that I didn't even want to "serve" myself! I ate what wasn't healthy, or I let my stomach get so empty that I'd get literally sick with hunger, and then eat whatever was convenient in order to not feel sick anymore. Usually it was whatever I could unwrap and eat, or pop into the microwave and stuff into my face with the barest minimum of preparation time and effort. This leads us directly into. . .

Martyrdom

If you're the cook, and you already have enough to do with the household and probably an outside job, you may set aside your needs because it's that much more work in shopping, preparation and cleanup and you already resent all the work that you're doing. Maybe you feel that you *are* serving yourself, in saving yourself from that extra work. You're suffering because you're giving your all to your family.

There is a lot to be said for the "benefits" of being a martyr. You can get a lot of attention and pity if you set aside your own needs for the benefit of others. But don't you sort of feel resentment for people who martyr themselves for your needs? Sure, it's nice to receive the benefits of their martyrdom, but who needs the guilt trip that automatically comes along with it? Do you want to be resented by those for whom you martyr yourself?

Being a martyr is a waste of time. Others resent you and you don't get what you want. Sounds kind of silly when you look at it that way, doesn't it? How about if, instead, you only do what you can, time and energy-wise, and let your family pick up the slack?

I know, I hear the screams, "How am I supposed to get them to help? They won't lift a finger!" You can just plain refuse to do any more than you're able. So the house gets messy or they don't have clean clothes. Where in the rules does it say that YOU have to do it all? If you go on strike, they aren't going to have a lot of choice are they?

If you're in a situation where you literally are the only person who can do it, then you seriously need to ask for help whether it's from family, friends, your church or community, or from Spirit. All of your arguments why you can't ask for help are just limitations you're imposing on yourself. Life really doesn't need to be so hard. And if you don't ask for help, you probably won't get it!

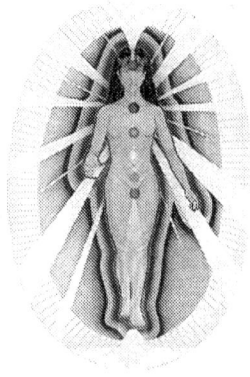

THE SCIENCE OF SHAPE SHIFTING

Junior High Science

It starts this simply: junior high science class. My science teacher, Mr. Messick,[35] stands in front of the class with a model of a molecule. It actually looks like Tinker Toys, except the sticks are connected by colored balls instead of Tinker Toy connectors. Each connector ball represents one atom and the color represents its type. He takes two blue atoms of hydrogen and joins them to one red atom of oxygen—H_2O. Blammo. Water. I don't get how, but okay, I'll take his word for it and memorize it so I don't flunk the test later.

Then he holds up more models, but these represent atoms. These have a nucleus—a center mass of energy made of protons and neutrons. Similar energy particles, electrons, are whizzing around the nucleus as though they're planets orbiting their sun. The atomic number, which is the number of protons, is what decides whether it's a hydrogen or oxygen (or whatever) atom. When atoms combine with enough *like* atoms, they form a quantity of a specific element that is perceivable to us.

[35] Shout out to Gary Messick and his partner in crime, Dave Habig, at Blackhawk JHS.

In addition, the rate of speed at which they vibrate (established by temperature) determines whether they're solid, liquid or gas—ice, water and steam are all H_2O. So far, so good. I understand him.

Now he says that the space *between* them, in relation to their size, is mind-blowingly large, like the amount of space between the planets and the sun. We can't even fathom the reality of it. The nucleus of an atom fills less than one billionth of its volume. If the nucleus were as large as a marble, then the atom itself would be nearly a half a mile across. In addition, none of this stuff is solid. It's all energy and emptiness, but it makes solid stuff. Our bodies are made of zillions of these energy blips and empty space. So is the book you're reading. So is the air between you and the book. The air itself is not empty space; it's thick with atoms that contain *real* empty space.[36]

Ready to blow your mind?

Since an atom is similar to the solar system, with thingies orbiting their sun, who's to say that our solar system isn't actually an atom? We might be living on an electron zooming around our nucleus, the sun, in an atom in the thumbnail of some unimaginably large creature. We can't see the creature or that we're in a thumbnail, because the space between us and other atoms is so vast that we can barely see *them*, much less the creature we make up.

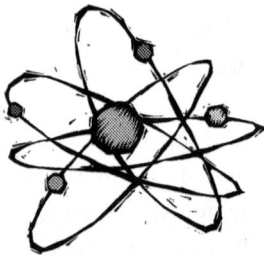

On the flip side, look at your thumbnail. One of the atoms within that thumbnail might just be a solar system, in which is an electron, upon which some teeny, weeny, itty, bitty little creature is reading a book, *completely* oblivious to your existence. I wonder—if you smashed your thumbnail with a hammer, if they'd feel an earthquake or tidal waves, or even

[36] And whatever *that's* filled with!

changes in their weather patterns. Wouldn't it be funny if they ran around blaming it on aerosol cans? In the meantime, it's just you cussing and swearing and holding your thumb, looking for something to blame it on!

How amazing is this? These little blips of energy and space—nothing, basically—create everything. These infinitesimally small electrical waves in oceans of emptiness work together to make solid, liquid, gas and the ethers.

There is no emotion involved for the atoms. They just do what they're drawn to do, go where they've been magnetically pulled. The active, aggressive waves move across and play against the receptivity of the dark emptiness. It's the ultimate yin/yang. If you can wrap your mind around that, you understand the meaning of life. It just *IS*.

What's the point of all this? To remind you that we're not as we seem—we're not the overweight body we belittle when we step out of the shower and see it in the mirror. We really are unfathomable numbers of atoms. Yes, you. This isn't just stuff to remember for a science test. This is the "real" world.

We are bazillions of whizzing thingies with massive amounts of space between them. It's a wonder you can't poke a hole through yourself with a wooden spoon handle (except that a wooden spoon handle is dull and is of a similar enough density to us that it won't go through us easily—you'd have to press pretty hard. A knife, on the other hand, is much more solid and sharper, so it would part your molecules more easily).

Now, imagine a thick cloud of dust. Then imagine that all the dust in that cloud, if it was all captured and compressed together, if its shape were shifted, would probably only make a small dust ball. There would still be errant dust flying around, but the ball is solid. What makes you different from the air around you is that you're a more condensed cloud of dust.

Let's hold that picture of ourselves for just a moment and move into another aspect of this energy stuff.

This may sound obvious, but think about it: *everything is made of energy*. We may know this as a phrase, but have you ever *really* thought about that? Everything that *is* (everything that we know of, that is) is made of energy. Everything. Solids, liquids, gasses—energy. So are television transmissions, radio waves, microwaves, x-rays—energy. Lipstick, fax machines, asphalt, construction workers—all energy. If this hasn't sunk in sufficiently, look around you and realize that everything you see, hear, smell, taste, touch, *sense in any way or not*, is energy. I don't want to beat a dead horse (which is made of energy, by the way), but this is an extremely important point to fully grok[37] before we go an inch further.

Once you've got a sense of the pure energy that surrounds you and *is* you, notice how the energy itself is neutral. It has no feelings, no judgments, no good, no bad. It's waves and empty space. It just *is* and it *is* every thing. I'm going to be repeating this phrase (which is energy as well) often because it's the key to understanding shape shifting. *Energy itself is neutral. It has no feelings, no judgments, no good, no bad. It's waves and empty space. It just is and it is every thing.*

Experiment time!

Let's make a Jell-O® parfait.[38] You have your parfait glass and your different flavors of Jell-O (energy, as well), mixed and ready to pour. You pour an inch or so of your first flavor in the glass and put it into the fridge to set. After a bit, go check on your Jell-O. It seems set enough to move on to the next flavor. You pour the liquid into the parfait glass and notice that, although the bottom layer is holding, the warmth

---

[37] For those of you who just said, "Huh?" I recommend the book *Stranger in a Strange Land* by Robert Heinlein. The word "Grok" is coined in this book and is meant to describe a sense of all-encompassing understanding of a concept with every fiber of your being. The reason I use it here is because it really says it the way I want to say it.

[38] You don't have to really do this, but imagine that you are following the instructions as you read.

of the new layer is melting just a touch of the cold layer and they're combining just a little bit. No problem though, because it's just a teeny bit.

Follow this same procedure for the remaining layers and chill until it's firm. (The process of chilling is energy. Did you know that? I bet you did.) Now hold your nifty parfait up to the light and see how beautifully Jell-O sparkles and how yummy it looks. Then notice that, even though there are many separate layers, they are all Jell-O in the end. In fact, there really isn't any separation between the layers because of that melting thing they were doing. In essence, this parfait is just one piece of Jell-O. If you tried to pull the layers apart now, it would be difficult because now they're all the same thing. The only thing really different is the slightly different vibration that allows the color to be different, and another different vibration that changes the flavor. But those differences aren't large enough to make a noticeable distinction in the vibration of the layers. The layers can't tell the difference because there is no separation. Even at a molecular level it's all atoms and energy and space. Therefore, the bottom layer is connected through the others to the top layer—it's one.

Let's go one more step. At some point during this process, while the different colored Jell-O layer molecules were saying hello to each other and sinking into each other's easy chairs, the peripheral Jell-O molecules were cozying up to the molecules that make up the glass (also energy). Now, they may all be energy, but that doesn't mean they speak the same language, or vibrate at the same rate of speed. However, that doesn't mean they can't communicate—they just won't be able to blend as well. So at the molecular level, the Jell-O and the glass are rubbing elbows—they're just not linked.

Stick a spoon (energy) in that glass of Jell-O (energy) and leave it there for a minute (energy). Now the spoon molecules are connecting to the Jell-O molecules, which are connected to the glass molecules. This means that the *spoon* molecules are connected to the *glass* molecules, *through* the Jell-O

53

molecules. If you still have your hand (energy) on the spoon (energy), then your molecules (energy) are connected to the glass (energy) through the Jell-O (energy) as well. In fact, your hand is connected to the glass through the air, or whatever else is nearby. It's one big electrical cloud of dust. Some parts are thicker than others, but a dust cloud just the same.

Any questions so far?

(Yes! What does this have to do with me being fat?)

We're getting to that, my little dumpling.[39] Patience. Anyway, you really have to grasp what I'm saying so far if you're going to grok anything that follows. So if you don't get it, go back and read it again. You have to know this stuff so well that you get tired of hearing it. That's why I keep pounding the point home that everything is energy. You truly must shift your thinking to this realization if you're going to shift your shape.

The Essence

The phrase "A fish out of water" describes someone who is out of his or her element. Say you're a fish (*I'm a fish*), and you're just living your life, eating plankton, going to school (*booooooooo*) and pooping where it feels right. As a fish, do you ever give any thought at all to water, the stuff you're moving through? That liquid that holds you up? How do you keep from plummeting to the ground? How does food just float up in front of your mouth like that? *What is this stuff???*

Doubtful. You're just living your life, eating plankton, going to school, and pooping where it feels right.

That's how we live in our atmosphere—living our lives, eating burgers, going to school, and pooping where it feels right. We really only notice the atmosphere when someone has fouled it up (no, I'm not making another poop joke[40]) or if the weather changes. But if fish can't see that they're in water, then what if we can't see what we're moving around

---

[39] Not a fat joke. Just a cute phrase.

[40] There are enough poop jokes in the world as it is.

in? The air has substance. It's just not something we can easily sense, just like fish can't really sense the water that surrounds them.

Let's go back to the Jell-O now. Your hand is connected to the glass through the spoon and the Jell-O. The fish is connected to the mermaid through the water. You are connected to me through *our* atmospheric connection. You are energy. The air is energy. I am energy. I am therefore an extension of you and vice versa. I am he as you are he as you are me and we are all together.[41]

> **Energy itself is neutral. It has no feelings, no judgments, no good, no bad. It's waves and empty space. It just is and it is every thing.**

Stay with me on this. If you are energy and I am energy and the air is energy and the fish is energy and the poop is energy and the Jell-O is energy then it ought to be pretty clear by now that *every single thing* is energy and *every single thing* is connected. *Every thing* is *one* huge thing: a sea of energy. Some spots are denser than others, but they're still part of one big thing. And *energy itself is neutral. It has no feelings, no judgments, no good, no bad. It's waves and empty space. It just is and it is every thing.*

Imagine that the air around you is very thin, crystal clear gel that you are able to breathe and easily move through— you're surrounded by Essence. Your body takes what it needs to sustain health from the Essence, and expels what it no longer needs. If you move your hands through it, you can feel its Essence. If you move quickly, you make a breeze— displaced air. And if there's something to be displaced, then there must be something of substance there.

Since this Essence is all around you, and since this Essence is made of energy, then doesn't it make sense that **you are Essence** too?

---

[41] *I am the Walrus*—John Lennon and Paul McCartney.

We are concentrations of Essence—of energy—so intense and so powerful that we actually have thought process and solidity. Think of carbon being compressed so hard that it becomes a sparkling diamond. We also have the "spark of life" that comes with an animated, living, thinking body.

One of the most important aspects of being human is that we have a personality, or the ego, which defines us as physical, *separate* selves. We are, however, still a part of the sea of every thing that is—we simply *perceive* ourselves as separate from others because it's one of the laws of physical reality. The world *as we know it* couldn't exist without separation.

It can be hard to imagine what I'm trying to say, since it's still not completely understood by mankind. We don't have the language yet to express the reality that exists outside of our physical world. Therefore, we have to rely on analogies in an effort to grasp a clue of the greater truth.

Picture yourself floating in a massive expanse of Essence. The expanse is so wide and deep that you can't see the edges. You're just a piece of glitter, a spark of life—conscious thought. The glitter (you) is made of the same energy and space as the Essence that surrounds it—it's just vibrating at a different rate—a slower rate than the Essence around it.[42] A tiny ball of vibration begins to form and slowly grows because the edges of the ball are jostling the Essence around them, which in turn slows its rate, which then changes the Essence around them.

This is basic creativity—Creation 101—taking a thought and molding and forming it. Now, going back to the concept that everything is energy, and that we are all one huge thing, it would make sense to say that even *god* is energy and therefore we are all god—the body of god.[43]

---

[42] The more solid a thing is, the slower its vibration.
[43] Look! I said that and wasn't hit by lightning!

This is what god does—it creates. It uses Essence—its body—to form whatever it thinks of. Its thoughts are those sparks of glitter that grow in the Essence.

Since god energy is the source of every thing[44] and it uses its spark of life to create, then when it sends another spark of life into the Essence as a seed of itself, whatever life form springs from that spark is a generator of creativity as well. It's a mini version of god that will shed seeds of its own, which will shed seeds of their own, etc., all within the Essence

How we create with thought

Life is created by our thoughts. Thought is *totally original*—even if your thoughts are a take-off on someone else's ideas, they are coming through the filter of your personality and so therefore cannot be exactly alike.

Thought is also *measurable* energy waves. In a process called biofeedback, thoughts have been shown to physically change the body, to change its temperature, and to relieve pain. Thought *is*. Thought has *substance*. **Thought hardens the Essence.** Yin plays against yang to create solidity. Thought is the first tool in shape shifting.

When you think, you send energy waves into the sea of Essence, like ripples on water. If your thoughts remain the same—when you focus those thoughts—the wavelengths remain the same. The vibration remains the same. The Essence hardens into the form that those vibrations create. Your shape is shifted.

The vibrations you send out if you say, "I'm a disgusting pig" are rippling and hardening the Essence. And if you think this sort of thing about yourself ALL THE TIME, the Essence just follows directions. Essence is energy and *energy itself is neutral. It has no feelings, no judgments, no good, no bad. It's waves and empty space. It just is and it is every*

---

[44] Until we learn differently, the buck stops there. Who knows where *it* originates?

thing. If you insist that you're a disgusting pig, that's fine with the Essence.[45] That's the shape it shifts you into.

As Neale Donald Walsch says in *Conversations With God, Book 1*, "Like energy attracts like energy——forming (to use simple words) 'clumps' of energy of like kind. When enough similar 'clumps' criss-cross each other——run into each other——they 'stick to' each other (to use another simple term). It takes an incomprehensibly huge amount of similar energy 'sticking together,' thusly, to form matter. But matter will form out of pure energy. In fact, that is the only way it can form. Once energy becomes matter, it remains matter for a very long time——unless its construction is disrupted by an opposing, or dissimilar, form of energy. This dissimilar energy, acting upon matter, actually dismembers the matter, releasing the raw energy of which it was composed."

> **The vibrations you send out if you say, "I'm a disgusting pig" are rippling and hardening the Essence. And if you think this sort of thing about yourself ALL THE TIME, the Essence just follows directions.**

With this in mind, how can you begin to dissemble and recreate the shape you want to shift? What if you started thinking, "I have a beautiful body," instead? Aside from your first reaction, which would probably contain a word represented by the initials "B.S.," you could actually begin to transform the Essence into that beautiful body. However, you need to make this your predominant thought so it can work on the Essence, and that can be very difficult at first. You need to become *immersed* in your new thoughts.

---

[45] If the Essence talked, it would probably say at this point, "It don't make me no never mind." That is, if the Essence were a character in *The Beverly Hillbillies*.

You must become immersed because if you only think your new, healthy thoughts *some* of the time, your thoughts are scattered. If your thoughts are scattered, nothing really comes of good thoughts because the vibes are all over the place and they don't have time to harden. Majority rules though. Whichever thought has the most concentration wins. If it's not over half though, or there are several conflicting thoughts, you'll lean more toward one way than the other— whichever thought gets the most energetic support—and unfortunately that's usually self-loathing thoughts.

We, in our physical bodies, are mini versions of god energy, like homemade batteries compared to the Hoover Dam. The power of the god energy creates planets and waterfalls and miles-deep oceans and galaxies and all the other stunning natural phenomena. Humans, on the other hand, create Beano.®46

So instead of blasting universes into existence, we individually work on a much smaller scale, the maximum that our current energy level will allow—creating our own human lifetime, and people who've learned to harness their creative energy invent things.

In the lives that we create, we experience—both individually and collectively—an incredible array of colors and flavors, tastes and smells, pains and passions, losses and triumphs. Not a single life is the same, just like the individuality a snowflake. Every moment of every day changes our life and shifts it toward this shape or that.

Our reality is just a game. Where else can we play cops and robbers, spy vs. spy, cowboys and Indians? Where else can we be cast in the role of butcher, baker or candlestick maker? How else could we know what it's like to be Romeo and Juliet, Rogers and Hammerstein, or Sigfried and Roy?

We chose our characters and our scenarios. We go through life gathering tools, potions, and weapons. We battle giant shadows and save princesses. We collect hit points and

46 No offense to the Beano people. I'm sure it's a wonderful product.

gain strength for the next level. *We* make it happen. We make *our* characters grow, not the other player's.

Your thought process is what steers your life. You make decisions that take you in one direction and other decisions you might have made would have taken you in others—all of which would make tomorrow a completely different path and years down the road a totally different future.

Each of us is a part of the god intelligence, a seed planted here for growth—a piece of glitter in the Essence. We feel and experience as much diversity of life as we can so that the *god source* experiences all that can be created. *We are not separate* from the god source. We are its nerves, its sensation source. Just as the nerves in the body send feeling sensations to the brain, we send feeling sensations to the god energy, into the Essence. Each lifetime has billions of moments that each have their own "flavor." Those flavors combine to create the overall lifetime flavor, which, to the Essence, is only *one sensation* out of billions and billions possible.

Every experience that we send back to the god source makes it larger, more experienced and expanded, more all knowing. It is all knowing because it gets its knowledge from itself and its creative parts, us.[47] It's aware of it all, but doesn't prefer one to the other. It's all good.

But what makes *us* who *we* are, as individuals with physical bodies? It's our consciousness' experiences and energetic influences. Before we're born, we're that bodiless spark of life just floating in the Essence. If we desire to expand and adjust our vibration properly and in the right direction, through conscious thought, our vibe matches those of human kind. We shift into a human shape. Like tuning in a radio station—this vibe equals that radio station's frequency. If we were going into a different direction, we might have shifted into frogs, or even in another galaxy or dimension.

---

[47] Think about what IT thinks of as a source! Ow! Brain cramp!

Thinking yourself fat

We think about the way we are "supposed to look" and the way we actually *do* look. We think certain things about certain foods. We think those things because they are what our blank slates have been taught. If we lived in other parts of the world, we'd be taught differently and we'd then think differently.

Part of the problem is buying into the "supposed to look" scenario to begin with. We simply *cannot* look like another person. Period. Even identical twins aren't 100% identical. So in our striving to look like a model, when our body knows better what it is *really* supposed to look like, we create conflict in the shape shifting process. We hate our body for rebelling against what we're trying to force it to do.

If you can't seem to *make* your body look a certain way, no matter how hard you try, then chances are real good that your body isn't *supposed* to look that way. You blame it on bad diet and not enough exercise, but that is only a part of it, and a small one at that.

Look at all the different, healthy body shapes there are. Tall, thin, stocky, muscular, willowy, and on and on. They are healthy and normal. Please note, then, that the stereotypical model figure is only *one of many*. Some people naturally look like that. They don't have to try, they just do. Just like I don't have to try to look short and curvy. I just am, no matter how much I weigh.

But somehow the people with *that* body shape have managed to get treated better and are practically revered, so therefore many of us want to shift into that shape. Who doesn't want to be treated better for doing absolutely nothing? However, if your body is genetically designed to be something else, even when it's at it healthiest, then I can guarantee that you will never ever ever ever ever ever

EVER—no matter how much you diet or how much surgery you get—never look like that body shape.[48]

You can't change that.

So if you have one of those shapes that doesn't fit into that one desired mold, then you're going to have to just accept it and start to think of your shape as *just as good as* the desired norm—because there's nothing you can do about it anyway.

Now, this isn't just a self-esteem issue. It's a creative issue. By thinking of yourself as having an imperfect body, then that's what you are creating whether you are aware of it or not.

If your body is genetically supposed to look like shape "A," then your body knows that and is trying to maintain that shape. But then you come along with thoughts and demands for it to look like shape "B." And unless you have the power of a Master, it ain't happenin.' So what you're actually getting is a weird morph of AB. That's why you are struggling to reach that goal, because your body doesn't know what to do with the energy you're pushing on it, so it just places it in the most pleasing manner that it can. You keep piling more of it on, so it starts running out of places for the energy to go. Gradually it looks less pleasing. Not less pleasing as in "less like a model's figure," but less than pleasing for *your body type.*

Think of it this way: could you make your body look like one of the other, "undesired" shapes? Could you go from tall to short? No? Then why on Earth would you think you could change it into that model shape when your skeleton and muscles aren't built like that?

Take a look at your bone structure and the healthiest, most fit people in your family. See whose body shape you most resemble. That's your goal—not some swimsuit model.

For example, I'm about 5'2" (5'3" on a tall day). I have a sort of muscular build. My thighs are naturally heavy and

---

[48] At least, not until you reach Mastery. But part of reaching Mastery is releasing the need to look a certain way to please others.

powerful looking. I have great legs when they're toned. I have wide hips, an hourglass figure and a larger than average bust. That's what I look like whether I'm fat or thin, there's just more or less of me either way. So when I make the effort—through changes to a healthier mindset, diet, and more activity to look my best—I'm still not ever going to look like a supermodel. I will not suddenly grow taller and narrower.

However, I can still have a pretty cute little package. So that's the goal I need to keep in mind for myself. A cute little package. I can do that!

Here comes that obnoxious metaphysical leap of faith you keep hearing that you have to make. In order to attain "perfection," you have to know that you're "perfect" already. But until you *do* think of yourself as perfect you will never *be* perfect. It's the most annoying paradox known to mankind, but it's true. Creativity is in the NOW moment. In order for me to have a "cute little package," I have to know that I already *am* one.

> **This isn't just a self-esteem issue. It's a creative issue. By thinking of yourself as having an imperfect body, then that's what you are creating, whether you are aware of it or not.**

Break it down: grab the perfect image that you just discovered from a family member, the one that your body has a chance of actually attaining. Think of yourself as looking like that. Even with a lot of weight on you, you can at least imagine that, because it's believable to you that you can get there. You can easily see your face on that body.

Keep thinking of yourself like that, *being* that in your mind's eye, and you'll gradually begin to look like that. You'll find that you just magically start eating better. You'll start thinking twice about eating sugar. You'll start parking a little further away than you have to, or noticing that your butt is sore from sitting too much so you get up and move around more.

Makes more sense now, doesn't it? In fact, it's logical. The problem is that we don't think about our bodies with logic, we do it emotionally, with much weeping and wailing and gnashing of teeth. Fact is, our body can only have one genetic mold. It's up to us to allow it to be.

What we are taught about foods can affect us as well. If I think, "cake is fattening," then it's going to *be* fattening. I can try to tell myself all I want that it's not, but my ego is still going to *believe*, deep down, that it is indeed going to make me fat.

In addition, if you tell your spouse, your friends, or whomever, that you don't think it's fattening, they will likely roll their eyes at you. The belief is too deeply ingrained in our minds, our culture, weight loss books, plans and methods and our fat psyches. So this is a really tough row to hoe. It's not the cake that makes you fat. It's our collective belief that it will. A collective belief has massive amounts of energy behind it—millions of believers compared to one nonbeliever. It can be exceedingly difficult to get past it.

Some people (usually very thin ones) KNOW that cake is not fattening for *them*, so they can eat all they want and not gain weight. They will, however, feel rather ill if they do, so they don't eat as much of it. We feel sick anyway, so we don't notice when we've eaten too much of it. It just tastes too good to care if it makes us feel bad later. It makes us feel good now!

We even picture foods making us fat as we eat them. How many times have you heard the phrase, "It will go straight to your hips?" We KNOW that food sticks to us, so therefore, it does. "Why not, if I'm going to be fat anyway, I might just as well have that second ice cream cone and get even fatter." So we are *literally imagining* ourselves straight into tighter pants. This is where the point that thoughts are actually measurable energy becomes so incredibly important.

Biofeedback, as briefly mentioned earlier, is a scientific method of training one's thoughts to control body functions. You are hooked up to electrodes, which are connected to the biofeedback machine. It then graphs out the movement of various muscles that you are specifically working to control with your mind. Your job is to move the measurement needles in one direction or the other, or to keep them still, with only your thoughts.

If your thoughts' affects on your *physical* body can be measured by biofeedback machines, then it would stand to reason that your thoughts can easily control something as delicate as your cloud of dust—your *etheric* body, or aura—as well. In fact, it would be easier to manipulate your energetic field, because the molecules there are *far* less dense and therefore much easier to move, like waving your arm through a cloud of dust and watching them all fly around.

God

What's God[49] got to do with clouds of dust? Not much, actually, but I was hard pressed to come up with a good segue. I mean, how do you segue to God?

Anyway, many people believe that it's God's will that they're living the life they have. Misery is their lot in life. Maybe God's punishing them, maybe God's testing them. You might not even believe in God. Whatever the case, "God" may very well have a lot to do with why you can't gain health and why you're heavy to begin with.

If God is outside of ourselves, and it's "God's will" that we are heavy, then we might as well just give up and go eat some ice cream. But if God *is* us, and vice versa, then we have some say in whether we're heavy or not. We simply have to decide to work with that god-self to create some changes in our lives.

So we need to look at God in a different way. This is the hardest thing to get past sometimes when we begin this path.

[49] Remember that when I spell God with an uppercase "G," I mean the God of religions. When I spell it with a lower case "g," then I mean god source energy.

Our fear of pissing God off keeps us from stepping over that line into discovery that *our perception* of God may be wrong.

Your experience with God may be totally different from mine, but many of the people I've talked to do have a similar image. God was an old man in the clouds, who got his kicks from torturing people with tests and impossible rules to live by. A slight exaggeration, perhaps, but this is the message I got as a kid. Kids—blank slates—tend to hear what adults tell them and then add their own twisted fears and logic to the story. This is how I saw God. For example, the worst sin I could come up with for my First Confession was that I didn't clean my room. I was mortified that I was going to fry in hell for this horrible mortal sin against Our Lord.

In addition, God didn't like women much. After all, weren't we the ones who made poor little, helpless Adam sin? Aren't we the foul temptresses who ruin men's lives on a regular basis? Aren't we supposed to be subservient to men? Aren't our periods unclean, a curse from God for our curiosity? Aren't our bodies sinful, capable of driving a normally reasonable man simply *mad* with lust? And, isn't God a man? Think I'm exaggerating? I have one word for you: "burka."

Little wonder I rejected God as an adolescent.

As an adult, I finally thought that I'd look back into this God business, if for no other reason than this way I'd at least *know* what I'm rejecting, instead of just doing it as a knee-jerk reaction to the horror show that was church of my childhood. What I found was a whole new perspective on the concept.[50]

I never discounted the idea that some sort of god-being exists, because I've always felt that there is some sort of intelligence out there.[51] *Something* had to cause our existence; I just couldn't believe it was a man with a beard, a lightning bolt and a rather cruel sense of humor.

---

[50] I'm not claiming to have discovered anything new—it was just new to *me*.

[51] Actually it's "in here," but we'll get to that later.

During my angry feminist phase[52] I did a lot of reading on women's issues and eventually ended up looking into Goddess-based religions. The idea of a deity who was glorified for all the things I've been taught to despise about myself was very interesting.

However, part of me rebelled against a female Goddess as much as against a male God. How can the one and only force from which we *all* come only be one gender? It simply doesn't make sense. And if there were a gendered God (yang, or masculine energy), there would have to be a Goddess (yin, or feminine energy) to keep the balance. And if there are both God and Goddess, then there can't be *one and only one* force. Therefore, the one and only force must include both genders because God is supposed to be all things. Consequently, god is best represented by the yin/yang symbol—a circle that holds two equal and opposite forces.

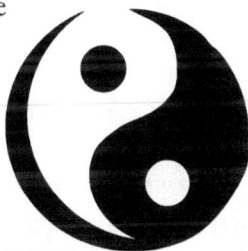

Since the most important part of shape shifting is connecting to your source of power, your god-self, then you need to be comfortable with it. If you, like I, see the word "God" as being a mean old man, then you sure as heck aren't going to be able to ask it for help and feel that you deserve it or that you'll get it.

Name your God

If any of this feels blasphemous to you, because your religion of origin taught you that thinking that you are part of God is a sin, then you can see this source of power as your Guardian Angel or something similar. Whatever works for you is best. You need to be able to feel and connect to the infinite source of power that *we all are*.

You can call it God, Jesus, Father, Mother, Spirit, Goddess, Yin Yang, All That Is, Universal Intelligence, I Am, Higher Power, Higher Self, Ra, Isis, or even Yippee Skippy.

[52] We all had one, didn't we? *Didn't we?*

The goal is that when you use that name it evokes a sense of connection to the awe-inspiring god/love/Essence—one that actually *likes* you and wants you to be happy.

Spend some time pondering what names suits you best. Get comfy with it. Curl up in your favorite blanket with it. Let yourself feel as though you're sharing hot chocolate with it. Whatever gives you the warm fuzzies is what we're looking for. You want to be able to feel wrapped in infinite love when you utter this name.

One of the best things I took away from the Goddess religion was magic, which is, in essence, metaphysics with toys and some really cool, dramatic rituals. Wiccans (witches)[53] practice a religion that includes the Goddess, and believe in our ability to manipulate energy and to create and manifest what we desire.

Once I came to this realization, I was synchronistically drawn to the concept of All That Is as a name for "God." All That Is was defined to me as the source of all power and energy in the Universe. Since, according to the Bible, we were created in God's image this means that we were created out of the same power and energy as that source, sort of like fingers on a hand. This means we are actually the body of All That Is.

Surrendering to God

Much has been said in self-help circles about "surrendering to God," or "let go and let God," and many other variations on the theme. The common understanding of that phrase is to give your problems to the old man in the sky and he'll solve them for you, if you will only believe in him. The same Christian concept is to accept Jesus into your

---

[53] Not all witches are Wiccan, but Wiccans are witches. Wicca is a branch of the Craft, like Lutheran and Methodist both hold Christian beliefs. And no, there is no devil involved. For more info, *Positive Magic* by Marion Weinstein is a great beginner's guide.

heart (or, open your heart chakra to unfiltered love energy, which is known as the Christ Consciousness).

This is a tough concept for an agnostic or atheist to wrap their brains around, and I had a lot of trouble with it as well. I wasn't about to give my life to God. He thought I was a second-class citizen! Why on Earth would I trust Him to take good care of my life? Surrender to God?!? No way am I waving that white flag! I'm not done here yet.

So instead I surrendered my ego's *concept* of God. And I also let go of the word "surrender," which to me means throwing your hands in the air and saying, "I give. Take me to your prison camp and do with my tortured body what you will." As Peter Quincy Taggart says, in the movie *Galaxy Quest*, "Never give up, never surrender!" My ego fought like mad, feeling all exposed and squishy, like a lobster that just molted.

> **Open your heart chakra to unfiltered love energy, which is known as the Christ Consciousness**

But if we look at it differently, we'll see that this is an amazingly helpful concept. What we need to do, instead of just saying "Uncle! Now stop hurting me!" is to allow the ego, or personality, to fall away. We are then open to Universal Intelligence. We can't do this all the time, because we need to function in the mundane world. We need our ego for that purpose. Our ego isn't *bad*; it's just sometimes misguided.

Inside the shell of our ego, which is nothing but energy anyway, we *are* Universal Intelligence. If we stop our ego from filtering it, we have access to all that is right for us. A friend of mine calls it, "returning to the sea of love." That sure sounds better than handing over the reigns of your life to some grouchy old fart who probably doesn't like you very much anyway.

I had a mind blowing experience with acupuncture many years ago that was actually a time when I "surrendered to

God," or allowed Universal Intelligence to surface, but I had no idea at the time that this is what I was doing. I only realized it years later, when I tried to deliberately do this "letting go" thing. My efforts to release my ego and open to this intelligence reminded me of what I felt then.

Acupuncture, in brief, is a method of clearing energy blockages in your body. It works on the theory of many energy lines (meridians) running through your body, connecting thousands of tiny energy points, or chakras, like power lines going from station to station. If one power station goes down, no power gets out to the areas it services and all goes dark. If that energy isn't reconnected, the meat in your fridge goes bad, you have no hot water, things begin to stink and bugs start to gather. That's a pretty rough analogy of how illness begins, but hopefully you get my point.

In addition to the acupuncture needles that he placed (and no, they don't hurt) I asked the acupuncturist for sort of a "psychic boost." He was a friend of mine, so he must have known what I needed. He placed one extra needle in the third eye area, right between my eyebrows. Then he left the room and allowed me to lie there, letting the needles do their work.

I really hope I can explain this in the way that it deserves, because it's the kind of experience that is difficult to put into words. The lights in the room were low, with incense and a couple candles burning. There was plinky New Agey music playing, so the setting was really cool and relaxing to begin with. As I lay there, just sort of drifting, not really thinking

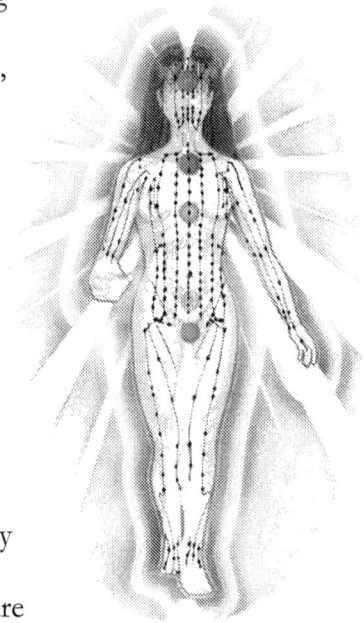

much, I began to see my body from a different angle. I saw the room get darker and darker, and a shard of light shooting out of my chest (heart chakra). It grew and expanded until it was shooting out of me in a straight line, from top to bottom. You've seen movies or TV shows where someone is welding through a bank vault door or a metal sheet of some sort. The light looked like the blowtorch flame when it finally comes through from the other side of the door and grows in size. It was cutting its way through me, cutting my body wide open from top to bottom, from the inside.

I "saw" my physical body fall to the sides, like I had unzipped my skin and taken off a costume. The blue light grew, continuing to shoot intense blue shards into the air around me. The energy built and grew and the light coming from inside me formed a line of brilliant white light along my spine. The room was filled with this amazing light and I just lay there on the table giggling and feeling totally peaceful. This was, without a doubt, the most awe-inspiring moment I had ever experienced.

I don't know what my friend saw when he finally came back into the room, but I must have looked positively goofy, with a big old dopey grin on my face. He asked, "How's it going?" with a big smile. I was worried that when he removed the needles the feeling would go away, and the blue lights had indeed dimmed and the lighting in the room returned to normal. But that awe stayed with me. I felt so large, and so good that I could still see a haze of blue light around me. I felt, "Wow! *This* is god!" All this without drugs!

This is when I realized what "love" energy is. Like my rejection of the word "God," I also rejected the word "love" as being sappy and phony. Love, to me, meant the kind of stories they tell in country songs. If you love someone, they'll leave you for their dog. Love was always something that hurt. All love stories involve torture and pain for the couple involved. An entire industry of romance novels revolves around the concept of love and pain. So like the mean old man in the clouds, who needs that kind of "love?"

But once I knew what the definition of "love" is—this intense feeling of "it's all good"—I then knew what "god" was. Suddenly the old expression "God is Love" made sense! I grokked it in fullness. Love, God, All That Is, Universal Intelligence, they're all the same thing!

What we need to do then is to really *love* our body. Allow it access to god, Universal Intelligence, love energy—see it as the Essence that it is. When you are accessing that love energy, or "surrendering to God," you're dropping the pretense that you're anything but a spiritual being that is made of energy—a light being. You feel like nothing can stop you and that all is right with the world. You only want what's best for your body.

Made in God's image

Let's back up for just a minute and look again at our current knowledge of basic chemistry. Everything that exists is made of atoms, which form molecules, which form mass. Atoms, which are made up of protons, neutrons and electrons, are energy. Between those atoms and molecules are huge amounts of space. So we are a mass of energy and space. We are, literally, an energetic mass.

God is an energetic source, and we were created in god's image. Our bodies are, in fact, solidified god. In that case, "God's will" is actually *our* will. What we have to realize then is who *we* are. We are not our bodies. We are part of god and we do have the power to create change.[54] We can and *do* shift our shape with every moment.

However, in order to create *healthy* change, we need to know what that means and what we're working with. We're working with food, fat, misery, frustration . . . you get my drift. This is what we focus on so that's what we get more of. However, there's no denying that we are dealing with some

[54] Actually, we can't really be "part of" god if we're all one thing. A *part* implies separation. It's our conscious selves that believe that we are separate and therefore able to be "part" of something.

concepts that have tremendous power in our physical world. They are . . .

Calories, carbs and the metabolism

We all know that a calorie and/or carbohydrate is what makes us gain weight, right? However, a calorie/carb is simply a measurement of energy. Nothing more, nothing less. Unfortunately, calories/carbs have been associated in our minds ONLY with getting fat. They might as well *be* fat for all we know.

Put the word "calorie" or "carbohydrate" in your Internet search engine and every single hit will have to do with weight loss and counting calories/carbs. That is a seriously heavy message. *Everyone* knows that calories/carbs make you fat.

Take a look at this, though. Except for the last definition for calorie (and not at all in the definition of carbohydrate), none of these even mention weight, and even the one does so indirectly!

Calorie *n.*

1. *Abbr.* **cal** Any of several approximately equal units of heat, each measured as the quantity of heat required to raise the temperature of 1 gram of water by 1°C from a standard initial temperature, especially from 3.98°C, 14.5°C, or 19.5°C, at 1 atmosphere pressure. Also called **gram calorie, small calorie.**

2. *Abbr.* **cal** The unit of heat equal to $^1/_{100}$ the quantity of heat required to raise the temperature of 1 gram of water from 0 to 100°C at 1 atmosphere pressure. Also called **mean calorie.**

3. a.) *Abbr.* **Cal** The unit of heat equal to the amount of heat required to raise the temperature of 1 kilogram of water by 1°C at 1 atmosphere pressure. Also called **kilocalorie, kilogram calorie, large calorie.**

   b.) A unit of energy-producing potential equal to this amount of heat that is contained in food and released

upon oxidation by the body. Also called
nutritionist's calorie. [55]

Carbohydrate *n*.
Any of a group of organic compounds that includes
sugars, starches, celluloses, and gums and serves as a
major energy source in the diet of animals; they are
produced by photosynthetic plants and contain only
carbon, hydrogen, and oxygen, usually in the ratio
1:2:1. [56]

If a calorie/carb is just energy, and we are energy as well,
then why does this specific type of energy transform into
solid fat, instead of just blending in like other energy?

My theory is that maybe we're missing or blocking
something in our energy field, or aura, that boosts the
metabolism. The metabolism, after all, serves to burn, or
transform, energy. A high vibration is needed to transform
the slower vibrating food. If we don't carry a high enough
vibration, then it's going to just sit there, like coal in a pile
waiting to be shoveled into the furnace. Perhaps our energy
fields aren't charged enough with the higher vibrational level
of love energy and Universal Intelligence, in the right places
that it needs for a healthy body, because our thoughts haven't
created it yet.

We need to raise our vibration—to replace the low-
vibration fat that we've created through our slow, heavy, and
possibly self-loathing thoughts, which bring our energy levels
way down. If the metabolism, a high vibration energy burner,
is simply the physical manifestation of love energy, then we
need to *love our bodies and raise our vibration*. And since love is

[55] *The American Heritage® Dictionary of the English Language,*
Fourth Edition Copyright © 2000 by Houghton Mifflin Company.
[56] *The American Heritage® Stedman's Medical Dictionary Copyright*
© 2002, 2001, 1995 by Houghton Mifflin Company. Published by
Houghton Mifflin Company

energy and calories/carbs are energy then we can replace the calorie/carb energy with love energy.

High calorie foods, ironically, are dense and thick, with a slower vibration because of their density—a lot of energy forced into a small space, so it moves more slowly. Low calorie foods are made of mostly water, i.e. veggies—not much energy and it's allowed all the space it wants, so it moves quickly. If you were to take low calorie foods and remove the water (no calories in water)—condense them— you would find that it takes a LOT to take up the same space as a high calorie food. In other words, it would take a huge amount of compacted carrots to equal the calories, space and/or density (not to mention yumminess) of brownies.

High calorie foods, being denser, vibrate at a rate similar to our physical bodies. Low calorie foods vibrate in harmony with our aura. They burn off more quickly because they are metabolized to correspond with the ethers surrounding us. The more fattening foods stay with the physical body. If you eat more of the fattening foods than the lower calorie foods, you will have more sticking to you and less will take its place in your field. A healthy balance is necessary.

It's possible that the specific range of love energy we're missing or filtering away vibrates at a similar rate to high calorie/carb foods—this translates physically into the belief that those calories/carbs will make us fat—they have power over us. If we had plenty of love energy in place, we wouldn't feel the need for any extra energy so we'd either burn it off, or not take it in to begin with! Since we're missing the awareness of this love, we are trying to replace it by eating certain types of foods—yummy foods that we looooove[57]— the kinds that are generally considered to make you fat because of their high calorie/carb content. We're bringing a replacement from the outside in, instead of realizing that it *comes from* the inside.

---

[57] Like Little Debbie® Swiss Cake Rolls. Mmmmmmmmmm.

The feeling that goes along with that heavy food is comfort: it will fill that empty space that you aren't filling with love energies. Ironically, fat is solid love. It is, after all, just solidified god. *Fat is how you love yourself. And we spend so much time hating ourselves because of it!*

If we're not burning energy and are allowing it to stay put, then we must need that form of energy to fill that space or void. We are missing a high frequency and replacing it with high calorie/carb foods . . . but we're misinterpreting and incorrectly processing that high level of energy.

I believe that our metabolism is actually the physical manifestation of how well we energetically love our bodies in that specific way. People who are thin have other problems to deal with that we don't have, so they concentrate their energies and tangled up problems in other areas of their bodies or lives. They love their bodies just fine, in the way that metaphysically and energetically would otherwise cause them to gain weight. We don't.

What's worse is that we're told "tough luck." That's the way your body works and you're stuck with it. No wonder so many of us feel cheated that they can eat anything they want and not gain a pound but if we walk *past* food it magnetically sticks itself to our asses. It's just not fair!

Here's the deal though. Universal Intelligence is not fair or unfair. It doesn't care one way or the other which way we choose to be. *Energy itself is neutral. It has no feelings, no judgments, no good, no bad. It's waves and empty space. It just is and it is every thing.* Why then would we be stuck with something that really is so unfair unless *we* chose to be?

It's hard to love your body when it seems to have betrayed you by getting fat. We look at our gut and think, "Yech!" We look in the mirror and sent hate vibes at our flabby selves. But ironically, that's what we've been taught that love is! It's all heartache and betrayal. You even buy your body chocolates when you want it to feel better. So you think you *are* loving your body, albeit in a weird kind of way.

If this is the case, then it shouldn't matter what or how much we eat, like thin people, as long as we first learn to train our thoughts. Sophia Loren explained it this way, when asked how she stays so shapely even though she doesn't diet, (and I'm paraphrasing here) "I just eat what I want and think thin." Easier said than done, I know, but remember what was said about "easier said than done" previously. Let's see if we can figure out how she does it.

Loving your body

The way a food makes you feel when you eat it can tell you how it is helping or hurting your body. If you eat an orange,[58] you feel alive and vibrant and zingy and all chock full of Vitamin C. You feel *orange*. You feel that zap of energy you get only from an orange. Oranges don't make you fat. How often do you really want an orange though?

Ice cream or chocolate, or pasta and bread make you feel full, solid, hugged and loved and all that warm, fuzzy sitting on Grandma's lap, reading a book on a cold winter day type stuff. That's fine, if you don't *need* the food to feel that way. But if it's the only way you get that feeling, you load up on those foods because that feeling doesn't last very long with this cheap imitation.

If these foods are your way of feeling that essence of love, then you're misinterpreting the energetic impulses in foods. They will solidify as *your body* if you don't fill that space with the same energetic vibe that it's replacing. If you had that exact same energetic vibe in place before the food, then fat would have no place to land. It wouldn't stay on your body. So, by filling yourself with that love, you can still eat the same kinds of food, but it won't stick to you. However, you may not *desire* those foods or large quantities if you have love energy in its right place.

---

[58] Unless, of course, you're allergic to oranges. Replace the word orange with something else that makes you feel up.

We are mistakenly replacing the missing energy, love of self, with physical manifestation. It feels real good when you eat something yummy, just as good as when you get a hug. So consider yourself hugged. If it helps, consider yourself hugged by God, or an angel, or a bunch of non-physical friends who want nothing more than for you to be filled with joy.

When you buy into what you've been taught, you keep your body's vibration down. In this way, you reduce the amount of love energy in your field. That's when you allow calories/carbs to shift your shape and become solid. By *believing* the incorrect information that you've been taught, you are essentially making yourself fat. So you need to pare away these issues as much as possible.

The power of your energetic field when it is expanded with love energy is a more powerful force field than the ego's muddy energy filter can be.

You see a model and you think, "I'll never look like that," and then feel lousy. That's your ego talking, trying in its twisted way to protect you from the harm you perceive would be done if you were thin. If you push aside your ego—which is your shell, your armor—you're going to feel vulnerable. But the power of your energetic field when it is expanded with love energy is a more powerful force field than the ego's muddy energy filter can be.

So instead of feeling all unprotected and needing your ego, picture the force field on Star Trek. Nothing can get past that—only attack from within can damage the Starship Enterprise. The more the ego is allowed to attack you from within, the more the damaging messages will eat away at your trilithium crystals.

When we love our body (or see it as solidified love energy), we want what's best for it. Normally that kind of statement would be followed by, "We give it the healthiest foods and exercise." And this is the kind of thinking that makes us feel even worse about ourselves. Of course we feel awful, if we give our bodies stuff that others say is bad for it. We don't blame them for judging us for being fat, because we think we brought it all upon ourselves with our constant pigging out.

Well, I don't know about you, but I really don't pig out. I don't eat more than most people I know, it's just that what I *do* eat makes me puff up like a blowfish. But is it the calories and/or carbs? Is it food reactions like Dr. Haas suggests in his book *The False Fat Diet*? Or my perception of what that food does and what I'm subconsciously trying to get from it instead?

Eat what makes your *body* feel good

Chocolate and many other foods make your *mouth* feel good when you eat them, but do they make your body feel good? Anyone who has ever dieted is familiar with the phrase "comfort food." It may make your mouth happy, but too much of it will make you feel sick. And many folks eat too much when it comes to comfort food. That's the point of it—to eat as much as you want and the heck with the bad guys who made you feel like you needed comfort food to begin with! Then when you feel sick as a result, you can say to them, "See? I'm sick now because of you!"

Certain foods act as comfort foods because they're rich and creamy and thick and fat and they just melt on your tongue. They give you a feeling of sensuous delight that you aren't getting elsewhere in your life. Or maybe they're crunchy and full of carbs, like chips or cookies. They help you to take out aggression as you chomp away. Sometimes it's just your favorite recipe that Mom used to make, and eating it now makes you feel like a kid again, before all the misery of adulthood came along just to piss you off.

Somehow, fruit and vegetables didn't make it into the comfort food category. They are low in calories and high in nutrition, and not very filling when you feel the burning hunger for comfort and self-pity. They sure don't make us feel warm and gooshy (unless they're in pie or something). Instead, they give us the essence of good health. Don't you feel it when you eat fruit or veggies? You feel that burst of "Wow! I just ate something healthy!" They make you want to jog around the block or do some silly aerobics tape, and who needs that? Doesn't sound like comfort to me! I can't *blame* anyone if I don't feel bad!

The essence of foods is their level of vibration, and each is as unique as snowflakes, fingerprints or atoms. Veggies and fruit, which are mostly water, aren't very dense so their vibration is very high. Fudge, on the other hand, is about as dense as food gets and the vibration is very low and sluggish. Thick, rich foods give us the essence of being still, of being bundled in a blanket and not having to do anything we don't want to do. They make us feel protected and loved.

I think this is why some foods make us fat and others don't. The number of calories/carbs is somehow connected to their essence. High calorie/carb, low vibe foods are the ones that allow you to feel still and cuddled. So if you're drawn to those types of foods, and too much of them, then you can reason that you actually need to **feel that essence**, not eat the food. Now it's time to find another way to fulfill that need. And if you want to gain health, you'll do it. No more excuses. Keep making excuses if you don't really want it to work—then you have deeper issues than weight. There's nothing inherently wrong with that, but you need to at least admit this is the case before you can begin to do any repairs. Otherwise you'll keep chasing an elusive dream and hating yourself even more for your "weakness."

We don't take more than the prescribed amount of medication because our body will react in a way that we didn't intend. If we take in more than the needed amount of any food, in order to get the essence of the food that we need, our body will react in a way that will give it either: heartburn, hives, upset stomach, diarrhea, or—of course—fat.

Back in the "olden days," food was considered to have certain energies, or essences, that were helpful for creating change. Nowadays, that type of thinking is dismissed in the mainstream as old-fashioned and superstitious. However, superstitions have a basis in reality or they wouldn't have been perpetuated for as long as they have. If there were no truth in it, it wouldn't be passed along. But back then, foods were eaten for prosperity, fertility and other ritual uses.

If it helps, think of food as a drug, as you would an herb or supplement. Your body only needs so much of a certain vitamin, herb or medicine. It also only needs so much of a certain type of food essence before you overdose. In his fascinating book, *The Magic in Food*, Scott Cunningham lists a multitude of foods and their essences. I'll list some common comfort foods and their corresponding essence, according to his book:

Bread—Protection
Pretzels—Protection
Rice—Protection
Potato and Corn chips—Protection
Tortillas—Protection
Garlic bread—Protection
Potatoes—Protection
Eggs—Protection
Chocolate—Love
Ice Cream—Protection, Love, Money

Do you sense a theme? All of these starchy and/or rich foods hold the essence of protection or love. Want to see a list of veggies?

Asparagus—Sex
Beans—Money, Sex
Beets—Love, Beauty
Carrots—Sex
Celery—Sex, Weight Loss

Cucumbers—Peace, Healing
Spinach—Money
Squash—Spirituality

Not much protection in that list. However, there's a lot of sex and beauty going on. Maybe we don't want these foods because we fear sex and/or being beautiful. His book lists many more foods that I couldn't possibly include here, so you may want to pick up a copy.

One night I was watching TV, and mindlessly eating sunflower seeds. Suddenly I realized that I had just eaten a fistful of sunflower seeds without even tasting or sensing them in any way, other than to just chew a big old mouthful. It dawned on me then that it only takes a seed or two in your mouth to get the essence of the seeds. I don't need to eat so many to get this essence. Since I ate more than I needed to get the essence, the excess—which isn't valued—will do what isn't valued. It will turn into fat.

Guess what sunflower seeds correspond with . . . you got it, protection.

Chew on this for a minute: think of the kinds of food you eat, on average. How are they reflected in your shape? Do you generally eat rich, thick, luscious food? Look at your body. It's represented there. Do you eat light, healthy, low cal foods? Look at your body. It's represented there. What about hearty, sticks-to-your ribs foods? What about junk? What if there really was something to the phrase, "You are what you eat?"

I personally feel absolutely great when I eat a vegetarian-type diet, like sprouts, tofu, wheat grass juice, that kind of stuff. I also adore Indian food. When I eat this kind of diet I feel vibrant and alive, like I could jump onto the roof and fly. I can feel my cells singing. I can do anything and life is so good I might just explode from happiness. When I eat chocolate and sweets and other things like that, my *mouth* thoroughly enjoys the experience, but my *body* rebels later with blood-sugar reactions, fatigue and just feeling icky in general.

If you know you're going to go ahead and eat something otherwise, enjoy every single bite without kicking yourself. Savor every mouthful. Really feel how good it tastes. Don't just mindlessly stuff it down your throat without tasting it. Your body doesn't want it, your mouth does! Give it your *full attention* and be in the Now as you eat. Give the food as a gift to your mouth (because we already know that it's the mouth that craves yummy stuff. The body craves nutrients.) And know while you're eating that it will have the effect on your body that you allow it to have.

Food is one of the most sensuous delights a human can have. How many times have you said something you're eating is "better than sex?" So if you're going to eat for taste, enjoy it, damn it! Let the food roll around on your tongue and frolic and play.

I've found that when I truly savor what I'm eating, I don't eat as much of it. I don't need three pieces of cheesecake because I *tasted* the first one. If I inhale the first piece, then my mouth didn't get the benefit it was after, so I need another one to make it happy.

Perhaps, if you indulge your mouth once in a while, and know that you can do it again when you want, **without guilt**, it will shut up about wanting stuff that makes your body feel sluggish. The deprivation mindset is what makes dieting hard. You might even try to see if you really need to actually eat the food. Sometimes just daydreaming about, for example, taking a trip to Paris and eating ice cream and pears at a

> **Food is one of the most sensuous delights a human can have. So if you're going to eat for taste, enjoy it, doggone it! Let the food roll around on your tongue and frolic and play.**

sidewalk cafe works. Who knows, your daydreams may end up creating that reality!

Listen to your body and *stop eating* when you're full. Yeah, yeah, you've heard that too. If you try this, and know when you're full but still want to eat, ask yourself why. Do you feel guilty about waste? Do you feel that you must eat it all because it may be a long time before you can have it again? If so, you may just live within a "lack of abundance" mindset. Remember that the Universe has an unlimited supply for those who are open to it. Trust that there's more where that came from.

Do you keep eating when you're full because you want to deliberately make your body feel bad? Because that's what you're doing. Instead, if you're full of food, but still feel empty, try to intuitively discover what part of your body feels empty and why. Then try filling that empty space with some of that love-energy that you have an unlimited supply of. It's not hungry for food; it's hungry for the energy that it's missing. Your body will feel much better and you'll feel better about loving yourself.

So perhaps we can gather from this that if we eat the kinds and amounts of foods our bodies (not our mouths) need, then we feel our best and gain health naturally as a result.

The aura

As I've already beaten into the ground, we are energy beings. It's hard to believe sometimes because we see arms and legs, torsos, facial features, etc. We don't have wires or hardware, things we have come to expect to see when talking about energy. We do, however, actually have an energetic "skeleton" upon which our bodies physically form. Around that body is a fine energetic "mist," which is called the aura, or human energy field.

The aura is not outside of us, however. It's a gradation of energetic mass—a *continuation* of us, outside of the physical shell. Like a light bulb, the light comes from within but the bulb seems the be the end of the physical light source. In reality, the light goes on and on, to fill the area with its radiance in the same way our aura does.

Here's another example—a lemon is a solid thing made of atoms, molecules, etc. If you cut into a lemon, you release many of those molecules by breaking the bond between some of them. You can smell the loose lemon molecules.

However, you don't have to cut the lemon to "sense" the molecules. Just hold it up to your nose and there they are, outside of what we *see* as the end of the lemon. They remain lemon molecules until they join with other molecules, and rearrange themselves to conform into that other energy. The molecules that enter your nose eventually assimilate themselves to become part of your mass. Now they are no longer lemon molecules, but nasal passage molecules. They work their way into your body and become a part of you.[59]

> **The human energy field is its energetic template, even where it *appears* to be solid. It holds the memory of your perfect body within its DNA molecules.**

Our bodies are similar in that our molecules extend beyond our bodies. Since we have a greater energetic mass than a lemon, the extension reaches farther beyond us than a small lemon's does. Like the force of gravity, which grows larger with the greater size of a planet or moon, the energetic force of a solid object can expand further by size. Think of the Earth's atmosphere in the same way—the Earth's aura. The atmosphere reflects the Earth's relative health, just as ours does.

---

[59] Paradox alert! I previously said that the word "part" implies separateness. Our physical, conscious lives depend on *perceived* separateness for their existence, so in physical life, yes, there can be parts.

The human energy field is its energetic template, even where it *appears* to be solid. It holds the memory of your perfect body within its DNA molecules. It knows what your best is and it can be asked to bring it about. It can shift its shape if you only ask it to.

Remember that your molecules are surrounded by *massive* amounts of space, even the ones inside your solid body, and know that they can move and rearrange. Thoughts, which are energetic impulses (remember biofeedback?), can be directed toward the molecules and shuffle them about to arrange a new form. (This is the basic concept of manifestation, of creating your own reality.)

If your thoughts are directed at yourself, this shifting takes place first in your aura. It takes your thoughts as instructions and follows them if enough thought energy is directed that way. Eventually the thoughts become solid in your body. The more power behind your thoughts, the more quickly your aura will respond.

If they don't take those opportunities, then it takes much longer for the energetic shift to happen in the aura, because the message it's getting is "I want to be thin but I'm not willing to make any effort to get there."

The aura isn't "magic" though, any more than any other mystery of life is. You can't just think and expect it to change—at least not quickly![60] That's where many people get confused when it comes to metaphysical thought. They misunderstand and think that all they have to do is daydream and their dreams will come true, because that's what they think is promised. Thought creates reality and we live in a reality where you pretty much have to eat less junk and exercise more. So thoughts about a healthy body will lead you to situations that help you to become so—

[60] Unless, again, you've attained Mastery.

they don't do the work for you. They *begin* the process—thought, word and action.

People who have trouble gaining health aren't following through on their thoughts with action. Their thoughts toward a more perfect body *will* magnetize them into healthier situations, like a more active job or perhaps a new restaurant with healthier foods, or a bargain on a gym membership. If they don't take those opportunities, then it takes much longer for the energetic shift to happen in the aura, because the message it's getting is "I want to be thin but I'm not willing to make any effort to get there."

The argument I've heard from people is "What good is this positive thinking nonsense if I still have to work for what I want?" Well, you're thinking anyway, only your thoughts aren't positive! You're doing negative thinking, which lead to negative words and actions! You're having to work *even harder* than you have to if you switch your thoughts!

Your thoughts are creating your life already, whether you know it or not. You might as well learn how to think healthier and get great results, instead of self-loathing, working harder than you need to, and getting either *no* results or *worse.*

The chakras

The aura is said to be arranged into different levels, each corresponding with different emotions and areas of the body. Each level has a corresponding energetic vortex, aligned along the spinal column, which also corresponds with those emotions and areas. These vortexes are the chakras that you've heard about and they exist whether you believe in them or not. Modern science is finally able to document this.

The New Encyclopedia Britannica[61] defines the chakras this way: "The chakras are conceived of as focal points where psychic forces and bodily functions merge with and interact

[61] Vol 3, 1993, page 58

with each other." Those "psychic forces" are the thoughts, the energetic impulses that we're talking about.

The first chakra, the root chakra, is located at the base of your spine and corresponds with the lower part of the body and the first layer of the aura, the one closest to your body and the densest of the layers. It corresponds with the most solid aspects of your physical body and is the foundation for mental and emotional health. It also connects to your will to live and your ability to give life your all. Its color is red.

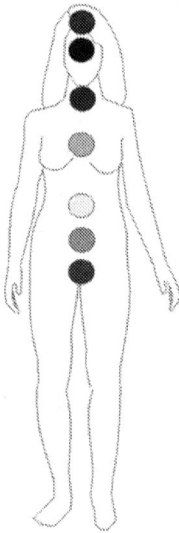

The second chakra, the sacral chakra, is located just below your navel. It corresponds to the sexual organs, bladder, bowel and lower intestine and the second layer of the aura, which is less dense than the first. It resonates with our relationships with others, with money and our creativity on a physical level. For women, this chakra is connected to our femininity, and for men their masculinity. If it's not functioning properly, it can interfere with your self-esteem and your sex drive. Its color is orange.

The third chakra, the solar plexus chakra, is located just below your rib cage. It corresponds with the stomach, upper intestines, liver, gallbladder, pancreas and the third layer of the aura. This is the center of our personal power, of honoring our self. Issues about one's appearance are located here. A strong third chakra will manifest strength of character, inner power and self-esteem. Its color is yellow.

The lower three chakras all relate to the physical body and the physical world. As we move up the spine, they become more etheric and thought connected.

The fourth chakra, the heart chakra, is located in the center of your chest. It corresponds with the heart and circulation, breasts, lungs, shoulders, arms, hands and diaphragm and the fourth layer of the aura. It acts as the connection between the lower, physical chakras and the upper, etheric chakras, blending the energies of both so they can work together. This is the center through which we feel and access love energy. This is also where we connect to "God." Its color is green (pink is also sometimes associated with the heart chakra).

The fifth chakra, the throat chakra, is located at the base of the throat. It corresponds with the throat and the organs within, the esophagus, trachea and the teeth, jaws and mouth and the fifth layer of the aura. This is the center of will and speaking your truth. It is also the center of personal responsibility and not placing blame elsewhere for creating what has occurred in our lives. We make our own decisions and keep our word. Its color is light blue.

The sixth chakra, the "third eye," is located in the center of your forehead just above your eyebrows in line with the pituitary gland. It corresponds with the brain, pituitary and pineal glands and the ears, eyes and nose, and the sixth layer of the aura. It is through this chakra that we visualize and access our intuition. Mental concepts are also worked out through this chakra. Our mind is connected to this chakra, the chakra of wisdom. Its color is indigo (or violet).

The seventh chakra, the crown chakra, is located at the top of the head. It corresponds to the energy that fills the spaces between the physical molecules in your body, the energy that activates life, and the seventh layer of the aura. This energy, which is spirit, is plugged into our bodies at this chakra. Our individual spirituality originates here. It is diametrically opposed to the root chakra, on the opposite side of the body, where one relates directly to the physical and the other relates to the energetic—both need to be present and to work together in order for things to run smoothly. Its color is violet (or white).

This information is useful when you look at your behavior as clues to the weight loss mystery. For example, I discovered that I put all my attention on my upper three chakras, devaluing the lower three—the physical world chakras. That was happening when I refused to do housework because I'd rather "think" like "men get to do." And my **body** suffered for it. I got FAT in the area of the lower three chakras!

The physical enjoyment of eating and sex were about the only physical things I did. I didn't realize that the lack of balance, of yin-yang, was part of my weight problem. By working to assure that my chakras were balanced I was able to more easily move into a mindset that allowed me to exercise.

Now what?

With all this in mind, it's easier to understand how we are indeed an extension of god, or Universal Intelligence. This intelligence is the source of matter, life, good, bad, up, down, All That Is. You can call it what you like, but it's *all* the same thing. It's all just energy, when you boil it down. [62]

So, if our body is energy, then fat is just energy, not a punishment from God. It's a manifestation of your thought energy into your physical body. What we need to do now is figure out which thoughts and energy have caused the physical manifestation of that fat. The problem is that it's not usually a conscious decision to become overweight. I don't know anyone who sat down one day and decided, "I think I'll grow my body into a shape that I will eventually detest." It's our unconscious thoughts that bring about the physical manifestations and with unconscious thoughts come the subject of the next section—emotions.

[62] I love footnotes.

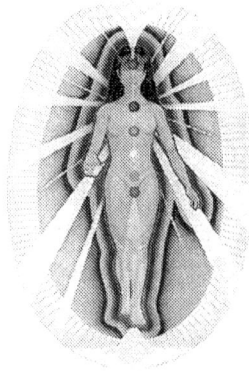

EMOTIONS

The ego

Our personality, or the ego, is what *defines* us as physical, separate selves. In the same way that our body is the *physical* translation of our energy field, the ego is what our energy field translates into *emotionally*. It's just as real as our bodies—it's simply another dimension of our energetic being, one we can't see or measure so it's hard for us to conceptualize.

It's one of the frameworks that our life is built on. It is the magnetic, energetic vibration that attracts similar people and needed experiences. It attracts what we do and see. It's made of Essence just like everything is because it's energy.

The ego is the filter through which we see life. It's the magnet that attracts what our thoughts magnetize. It's a wall of slowed-down-vibes between our god-self and our conscious self. It is energy, too. And *energy itself is neutral. It has no feelings, no judgments, no good, no bad. It's waves and empty space. It just is and it is every thing.*

If we didn't have the ego, we couldn't be solid because its energy pattern is what slows us down enough to *be* solid. However, with the ego filter in place, we can't access knowledge that lies on the other side of the wall without some work to speed our vibration.

This doesn't mean that we're stuck here in the slow, heavy sludge of our physical vibration. We do have the ability to see past it and to work with energy beyond it on either side. However, you have to work at it. You have to rise into the faster vibe.

We all know it's easier to go downhill than up. It takes much more energy and effort to take off in a jet than it does to land, or to ski or ride a bike downhill. Speeding one's personal vibration takes more effort than just maintaining its current level. Many times we don't bother because we don't know that we can!

A huge portion of our physical life is aimed at teaching us that we can't, that we're messing in God's business. Many religions teach that it's blasphemy to even dare to define god. Getting beyond that scare into self-discovery is a big hill to climb.

That's why it really helps to look at life from this direction, that of energetic process. *Energy itself is neutral. It has no feelings, no judgments, no good, no bad. It's waves and empty space. It just is and it is every thing.* Note that there is no mention of God (capital "G") or Satan. It doesn't contradict or imply anything moral. It's neutral. And it just is.

Look at the personality as the mold into which we pour our perceptions. It decides what shape our life will take. If we have taken on the thoughts and personality of a bitter, lonely and angry person, then that's the mold into which all of our thoughts will pour. That's what is magnetized to us. All of our experiences will take the shape of this reality until we change the mold. This is why things work for some people but others, with the same effort, will fail.

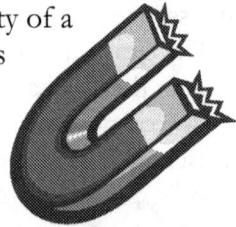

If our mold is that of a fat person, we can't stay on that "diet." Somewhere our filter says "fat" and it knocks us off track every time. It will continue to do so until we make the decision to change, and make that energetic shift. Until we do, we will continue to cry and to hate ourselves and to feel awful when thin people are around, looking so much better than we feel we look.

Those self-judgments, negativity and lack of resonance with healthy Essence are the basic symptoms of energetic imbalances. We need to work with the ego to change our magnetism. And it's mandatory that we do so with this thought in mind: *Energy itself is neutral. It has no feelings, no judgments, no good, no bad. It's waves and empty space. It just is and it is every thing.*

The word "ego" is somewhat misunderstood. We say that someone has a big ego if they think highly of themselves, or we feel that we are being "egotistical" if we talk ourselves up. However, there are several facets to the ego. It serves many purposes, some of which we've evolved beyond—just like the appendix, which used to serve a purpose when humans ate a caveman diet, but is no longer all that necessary.

The ego is the part of us that feels fear. It keeps us from being hurt, by "protecting" us from failure. Imagine a wire-stripper being used on your finger, ripping away the flesh and muscle, just leaving the bone exposed. That's what the ego is afraid of if it's stripped away—exposure. Once it's gone, it thinks your exposed core is going to be as sensitive as that stripped bone

The ego defines us as a personality—it's the skeleton upon which our experiences are hung to form who we are. Since we don't usually spend a lot of time picking apart and reality-checking everything that happens to us, there are a lot of misconceptions hanging around our psyches.

We react to things as a result of our experiences and not connecting to the god-self before we act. It's the ego that records what our blank slate is told and plays it back to us at a later date. You're told when you're young that you're good or bad, and the ego jots that down. Later on, it reminds you of what it's heard and then you use that information for decision making.

The ego doesn't know that "you're stupid" isn't the most helpful information you've received. It just stores it for future reference and reminds you later.

The ego is our survival instinct. The strongest instinct humans have is to survive at all costs. Fear of death keeps us from doing dangerous things, but it can also keep us from knowing our god-self.

For example, when I first began meditating and getting somewhere with it, I would feel myself disconnecting from my body. Part of me was really into it, thinking, "Wow! This is what they're all talking about!" But my ego was screaming, "Red Alert! You're dying, idiot! Pull back! Pull back!" My survival instinct won and pulled me out of what would later prove to be amazing experiences, once I learned to get past my ego.

It's the ego that stands between our god-self and us. This doesn't mean that the ego is an adversary. It's simply a part of who we are in the physical world. It's our definition. And it can be changed, once we're consciously aware of its presence and purpose. It can work with us if we choose. It can help us to shift our shape.

Depending on how often and strongly early messages were delivered, those changes can be easy to make or tremendously difficult. However, by using the power of your will, which is stronger than the ego, those changes are possible.

Truth

One reason that it's so hard to change our mold is that sometimes it *hurts*. Sometimes we go through ugly circumstances to get from one place in life to the next. And if those circumstances are part of, or even all of, what plopped us on the road to fat, then we're not in a very big hurry to think about those circumstances, much less examine them closely to rework them. Dredging up old, bad memories is not the most fun you can have.

However, from an energetic standpoint, it's helpful to at least go back and smooth out the energy that bumped you off track from a healthy, attractive body.

Going back and looking at the origin of the energy quirk isn't going to be anywhere *near* as painful as the original event. In fact, sometimes you'll find that what freaked you out then really wouldn't make you bat an eye today. It was just blown up because you saw it from a less mature perspective and couldn't wrap your mind around its meaning.

Your memory of any event is automatically distorted toward the way in which you have learned to perceive things. No one else will remember any event in the same way you do, because they have their own distortion

> **Resonating with the Essence is the way we're *supposed* to feel—when we're not filtered by our ego—and it's what we're shooting for in life.**

and filter. The actual, undistorted truth of an event can only be seen by someone whose filter at that spot isn't energetically (emotionally or physically) charged and/or blocked. In this case, seeing the truth doesn't hurt. Their energy isn't passing through a protective filter.

Think for a minute about how often you are actually happy—just content (which is truth vibes). You're not hungry or thirsty, nothing hurts, and you don't have to go to the bathroom. Life is good. Not very often, right?

Then think about a time that you just felt great. Even if it was 15 years ago and only lasted for a minute. Try to recall that bliss. Whatever was going on for you at that moment was in line with "god." That's just a glimmer of what true love feels like and that's what it insists on maintaining. If you don't flow with the Essence, it *will* insist and knock you around until you agree to flow with it. This is what causes what we call hard times in life. The further we go off track, the harder we get kicked in the pants to make us get back on track.

You're not resonating with love/god/Essence and until you do, it's going to *hurt*!

Resonating with the Essence is the way we're *supposed* to feel—when we're not filtered by our ego—and it's what we're shooting for in life: it's our goal. It's the heaven we pray for. It's why we go to church and volunteer with the Red Cross. It's why we play with puppies and squish our toes in the wet sand and eat chocolate. It just feels *so good* to be one with All That Is.

The ultimate in going with the Essence—having a connection to All That Is—is the orgasm. When we ride the wave of Essence, we can reach ecstatic heights and commune with god, with the Oneness. It's also why we do drugs . . . they vaporize the ego wall between consciousness and the Essence. Unfortunately, a huge portion of the Earth's population are so out of balance that they abuse these tools and cause them to be illegal for those who could responsibly put them to good use.

Pain lives in the aura first

Let me reinforce the points necessary for this specific concept, which will tie in together.

- We are energy beings made of love/god/Essence, in the love/god/Essence, and we take on solid shape and individuality through slower vibration, thoughts, experiences, and focused effort.
- Our solid being is nothing more than densely packed programmed energy, and as our beingness gets further from our center, less solid, our intelligence is still the predominant vibe until we have lost interest in continuing to mingle with the Essence. The energy outside of our solid self is still us, because it contains our version of the Essence . . . our energy field. This is the aura.
- "Pain" and "hell" are synonymous. Hell is the opposite of Heaven (God = Love). Pain is the opposite of resonating with the love/god/Essence.

Depression is pain—lack of conscious connection with the love/god/Essence. Physical injury is a lack of connection. Any time you feel pain, it's the opposite of love. Pain in your body is a symptom that something is wrong. So, if there is pain in your body or psyche (your thoughts—energy), then there is something energetically wrong. This can be fixed.

- The pain or discomfort you may feel while looking back and smoothing the rough spots is only energy and *energy itself is neutral. It has no feelings, no judgments, no good, no bad. It's waves and empty space. It just is and it is every thing.* If you don't go through this process, then the energy that was left behind during those circumstances, the energy that makes up your distorted memory (which is just a stuck thought) is going to fuzz up your aura with discordant energy.

If your aura is fuzzed up, then the energy that is your body will be out of alignment with your true essence. If there is discordant energy, caused by an uncomfortable event in the past, it's still hanging around in your aura because you haven't unblocked or cleared it.

It's just sitting there festering. If it stays long enough, with the focused attention on it, or dwelling on the pain, eventually it's going to become physical just because it's vibrating more slowly (by being conscious thought and in your proximity) and is being brought into your body. You're internalizing it and eventually you could end up with a disease or . . . fat. You have shifted your shape away from its most exquisite self.

So now we narrow down another cause of fat. Fuzzed up auras that need to be cleared of discordant energy.

We are, however, still a part of the sea of every thing that is. Therefore, our pain affects the collective whole. By healing ourselves, we actually help to heal all of humanity. After all, there is only One of us.

The power of collective energy

Let's step back now, just a bit, to the question of what are solid things and why do they look the same to everyone if we all create different realities. For example, Mount Rushmore looks like four presidents carved in a mountain to everyone with sight because we, as a collective, have agreed to a set of rules and structures to live by. This is why the oceans have a certain depth and breadth, and the definitions of physical life don't change very much from person to person. It's only in our own personal lives that we can truly make changes because it's in our own personal power to do so.

Universal Intelligence formed our playground Earth with so much intensity and focus, so strongly, and with its *massive* size, that we couldn't individually change its appearance if we tried. We simply can't pack that kind of energetic punch.

We do try, actually, but in such tiny ways that it takes an awful lot of *combined* human effort before our changes are noticed by the planet.[63] If, at that time, the changes we've made are unhealthy for the planet's beingness, it gives us a kick in the ass by changing weather patterns, or blowing its stack with a volcano or shaking us awake with an earthquake. It may even just start letting holes get punched in its aura.

It's almost as though we're fleas on a dog's back, and the dog will only really scratch if we cause a big enough itch.

This is not to say that I think disasters happen because "we cause them and are being punished." What I'm saying is that the energetic imbalance that we cause through our thoughts and actions has to be righted and sometimes the planet needs to seriously shift in order to balance it. It's our *conscious* misfortune if we happen to be there when it happens. *Unconsciously*, we are there specifically for that experience.

Since the Earth is such dense energy, we just don't have the ability to see where its vibrations begin and end while

[63] In fact, it took 14 years and over 400 people to carve Mount Rushmore.

we're in physical form. Our abilities in that way end the same way that our physical ears can't hear a dog whistle or in the way that our physical eyes can't see beyond ultra violet or infra red light, or even see the Essence. We just haven't learned how to stretch our senses that much *yet*.

We are, as a race, certainly growing in that direction, but it's a slow process. Therefore, what has been created as solid by All That Is *is* solid to us. Even if we try to destroy it, we're still left with visible or measurable signs that it's still here. And since we see Spirit energy's creations as solid, and we all have similar human perceptions (the same ranges of vibrations are visible, audible, etc.), we see solids as basically the same shapes and sizes, etc. However color blindness is one example of how varied perceptions can be.

(*But, I'm still fat!*)

Perhaps, but you're starting to see it differently, aren't you? Even just a little? Do you begin to understand why it's so hard to change your physical form without changing your thoughts about it first?

Desire

Desire is one of the first steps in creating. Desire is mandatory. It's not a sin to want. It's *NECESSARY*. If you didn't want or desire something, you wouldn't bother to get out of bed, much less draw breath.

Desire is one of the elements of life. Religions that teach you that desire is a sin just don't get it. People are told that it's selfish to want a different life, or to live the way they want to live. So they don't allow themselves to desire something better, and they create a reality of misery.

We're not selfish or vain to desire a better life or a beautiful body, if that body is a true representation of our ultimate essence. Human beings appreciate beauty, so why shouldn't you be able to appreciate your own beauty as yet another creation? It's something *you* created!

It's just a goal to create, and a reason to get up in the morning, just like raising a family or boating around the world. It's your desires that pull you forward. If you negate those desires you go nowhere fast and life is pretty gray. Anti-depressants have come in handy for a whole generation at times like these for people who aren't living the life they desire.

Since you've created your life and your physical self, you might wonder, "Why on Earth would I choose to be taught that desire is a sin?" We've been drawn toward human life for the varied experiences it offers and the endless opportunities to create. Our vibration is our individual waveform, unlike any other, like a fingerprint. In order to become physical, it needs to find parent waveforms whose vibes are similar enough for it to mesh with and create a new body for itself; otherwise there is just no match.

If you didn't want or desire something, you wouldn't bother to get out of bed, much less draw breath.

If one waveform that is enough like you becomes pregnant with another that is like you in other ways, that combination fits your energy well enough for you to move into that newly created physical form. Your body is truly a combination of your mother and father's physical energy. Your spark of life is the glue that joins the yin and yang of male/female energy, sperm and egg, and creates another human body.

This is what's meant by the sometimes-confusing phrase, "we choose our parents." It's not you in your body sitting on a cloud looking down saying, "Hmmm. I think Bert and Debbie would be good parents. I think I'll pop in," or, "I bet Tammy and Dave would allow me to be sexually abused. Let's try that!"

You, as intelligent life, choose to become a human on Earth at this time, place, and with these people because the vibe at that moment and space matches what you have created energetically and non-physically. These people, who match you fairly closely, raise you and that helps you to stay on that track that you've chosen.

Adoption could very well be caused by entities who change their minds about being together for life, and agree to go separate ways. Perhaps they only wanted to experience physical form together for a short time and were done with the experiment. Then they agreed to move on and new parents with the new vibe you're looking for are drawn to you and you to them. I imagine that's the same case with aborted babies or stillborn babies—that entity just wanted the experience of being physical for a short time in those circumstances and at that vibration. Maybe it's just using that vibration as a between-vibe bridge, to take it from vibe A to vibe C.

Blame

Our final "emotion," blame, is a waste of time. Even blaming ourselves isn't appropriate. We create what goes on in our lives. If we weren't in some way magnetically attracted to our circumstances, they would have passed us by and not stuck to us.

It's very easy to blame circumstances or other people when life is rotten. In fact, it's a way of life for a huge number of people. When something goes wrong, they immediately begin casting about for a scapegoat. However, it keeps them stuck in the pattern that created the disaster in the first place. Sometimes it just doesn't matter "who did it." What matters is how the situation can be learned from and repaired.

Blame negates the fact that we are energy beings and that life just is. It is what we make it and circumstances are in our lives because we attracted them to us. There is no blame. It just is. When you feel the need to point a finger, ask yourself what part you played, because you did play one. So if they are to blame, then you are to blame as well. Someone once said that whenever you point your finger at someone, you've got three pointing back at you. So when you point and say,

"You!" you're actually pointing at yourself saying, "You! You! You!" This leads beautifully to the topic of . . .

Projection[64]

In essence, we project—or blame someone else for—our negative attributes when we focus on "their" flaws. We see things in others that we don't want to see in ourselves. Another version of projection is when we mirror—or give someone else credit for—our positive stuff when we admire "their" good qualities. We see in them what we most want to be, but don't realize we already have.

A simple way to look at it is that life gives you feedback. Once you learn to listen to it, you can unravel problems that have vexed you for years. Paying attention to what you project is a way that you can see what your issues are, where your life needs to be healed.

We all have an interior reality, which is the life we see and create through our personality filter. Everyone lives his or her life getting feedback in one way, shape or form of that interior life. You can think of life as your laboratory.

The spiritual journey is about becoming inclusive, opening up to and owning all of the disowned parts of us. It is only through our wholeness that we can really thrive in the world. So we look to others to fill in the spaces we feel are missing. We admire someone's brains or beauty because we don't believe that we have them. We try to throw out the things we don't like and give them away to others. We see them as "stupid" or "ugly" because we fear we are those things or may become those things.

We're constantly projecting our material outwards. That doesn't mean necessarily that we have "issues" with it, however. You can tell it's an issue if you overreact, either

[64] This section was adapted from a class taught by Victoria Wilson MS, CCE, CHt, which was based on the work of Maria Von Franz, and an article written by Lisa Bonnice and Victoria Wilson about that same class.

way. If you feel, "This is the perfect person and I must be with them," or, "This person is the demon spawn from hell—get me away," it's an overreaction. Then you'll be safe in assuming that it's an issue.

When you stop to think about how complex we are, you may realize that projection is a gift straight from Spirit. It becomes the way that we know what to work on next. What we need is structures and boundaries so we can explore. That's where projection comes in handy.

Projection can be broken down into five stages, from a spiritual standpoint:

1. **We look around to find the perfect person to hold our projection.**

   One of the easiest ways to find out what issues you're working on right now is to make a list of qualities you want to find in a lover or mate. This is what is important to you *right now*. It does change over time. If life's been a drag, you're going to a want someone who's fun and playful! If you feel like you haven't been out with friends in years, you're going to think, "Wow, I wish I could find somebody to talk to! I want to find someone with a mind, and who's doing something with it." A lot of what you're looking for relates to what's developing inside you.

   Then you find someone who fits those needs and begin that honeymoon phase, which is wondrous—this person has got it all going on. They've got everything! That's Stage One. Stage One is finding the person to project on. So you're involved now and you're projecting and mirroring like crazy. And you're giving them credit for all these wonderful things that really began within you. They help you to bring these things out because they are someone with whom you can share.

2. **The projection begins to slip.**

   Eventually that person can't meet our needs because they've got their own life and work to do. We begin to see that the individual is something other than what we have imagined. We don't want to believe this so we make up stories and excuses. We've tacked this image, this projection screen, over them and the corners start peeling off. We run and get a hammer to tack it back on.

Then we begin making excuses for them. We say things like, "You know, he's a very sensitive person," or, "She was just tired." We make excuses for why they're not being who we thought they were. This begins happening more frequently, for longer periods of time, until eventually we move to Stage Three:

3. **The projection falls off.**

We are forced to see what is beyond the projection, the real person. At Stage Three we have a few reactions to choose from.

We may begin to feel hopelessly betrayed, "That bastard," or "That bitch! They weren't at all like they told me they were. They told me they were like this! How dare they!" So you can get trapped in the victimization process and feel betrayed. Then you'll go all the way back to Stage One with that same person, who is promising to be the way they were before, and then slowly slipping back.

Or you might start the process with a new person just like the last. That's why you feel like you keep getting involved in the same kind of relationship over and over again. What happens is you go 1, 2, 3, 1, 2, 3, etc.

The trick is to go on to the second choice after Stage Three. You can go on to Stage Four. That's when you recognize that what you've been projecting onto this person is what you'd like to become. It's recognition that you're projecting onto them the qualities that you'd most like to bring forward in yourself now. It's either that or regress backward to Stage One, feeling let down and betrayed, and the process begins again.

4. **We recognize that it is our own material.**

This is the stage of grief—grieving for the part long lost—grief over not truly seeing another for who they actually are.

If you were looking for trust in a relationship, it usually takes you into that pit of thinking that you've really been betrayed. When we're looking for somebody trustworthy, we're really looking to try to trust life again because it's become hard. So you realize that "I was really looking for it to be okay for me to be sensitive or trustworthy or fun." "I've been waiting for permission to have fun, and how long have I been waiting for somebody to tell me that it's okay?" We find that recognition of everything, that all the qualities that we're putting on that other person are the qualities that we're most wanting in *ourselves*.

Stage Four is challenging. It requires someone with a real adult perception. It's also the part of the spiritual journey that most of us struggle with because every one of us has free will defined ego. We have to realize that, "As long as I was projecting on that other person, I wasn't really seeing them." So there's sadness. If you stay with it you will move to Stage Five.

5. **Compassion and integration of the projection.**

Stage Five is the integration of these qualities. We have compassion for others and ourselves with similar issues. We begin to model the qualities that we once projected onto another. You embody them. You bring those qualities into your own life that you one time tried to find in someone else. As a result, you're going to find compassion for someone who's going through the same issue.

You can tell when a person has really worked through an issue because they have compassion for that issue. Once you've really dealt with your own weight issues, you'll be non-judgmental of people with the same problem because you know how paralyzing it can be. Someone who says, "Oh, I've been there. Toughen up. Work your way through it." is heading for 1, 2, 3. They haven't worked it.

Stage Five is freeing. You can look back and say, "That was worth it. That was incredibly worth it."

Once you get to Stage Five, you have new knowledge that will help you to solve further mysteries. We really are one heart, one mind. We are all learning to love all these different parts of the Oneness. That's not to say that you won't run across parts of yourself that are uncomfortable and scary. However, every single way that we can manifest is valid, including being heavy. It's simply a clue, pointing you in a direction to begin looking.

If we have a limited idea of what's okay, it's that limited idea that makes us control freaks. If we follow projection, it will consistently take us into being more compassionate and open. If you're compassionate and open, you can have a pretty interesting and mystical time.

You don't have to keep yourself within a projection that you don't like. You don't have to eat worms until you enjoy the taste. But what you need to be aware of is that if you don't own it, it will come up again. Until you clear the energy of this issue, it will keep coming back until you do. Hence, the inability to lose weight and keep it off. There is an issue that needs dusting off. With each projection that you deal with, as you own them and as you dig to find the core belief that has not served you, what you then begin to project is the direct opposite of the original projection.

When people don't work to consciously grow and understand themselves, they tend to draw a lot of people to them who play out the different issues they have been trying to stuff down. Life keeps insisting that we be whole. It stimulates our issues and limitations so that we will get past them, so we will address and heal them. Look directly at where your life sucks the most. That's where to work first.

Life only whacks us in the head with a board, though, when we don't listen to its previous nudges. Don't wait until a disaster has to happen for you to pay attention, like becoming morbidly obese or developing serious medical issues as a result of your weight. If you're already in that space, then you have an easy choice of where to work first.

Many times your inner adult is struggling with your inner adolescent. Your masculine is struggling with the feminine. The inner child is beaten up by the inner adolescent. Have you ever been in a relationship where you feel very deeply that you're persecuted and sad? You're probably polarized into a feminine child part of yourself, and that attracts bullies and tyrants. It actually *pulls* that out of others *and* out of us. If we don't have an external bully, we *will* bully ourselves. Do you say really cruel things to yourself? Bingo. We have all these different forces on the inside that can minimize and stop us from having a life that is fulfilling and has enough adventure, joy and creativity. We can be betrayed by parts of us that are there to protect us.

Let's say that you feel someone is talking down to you. You need to go back in time to find somebody else who used to talk down to you. While journaling ask, "Who else has talked down to me?" Very often it's the way we treat ourselves. By beginning to speak more kindly to ourselves, we will begin to attract others who do the same because that's what we'll be projecting instead.

People also project their issues onto you. If you can work through your end of it, and stop responding in the way they need, then they won't get the reaction they need to continue the behavior. They'll have to find someone else to project onto. It will be a different energy—your energy changes. Whatever their behavior is triggering in you, it's changing your energy. Your energy is shrinking and you're becoming the energy of a younger age, emotionally. Pay attention to whatever age you become, and that's a key, "How old do I feel?" The age you feel could be the age where it began.

Fear of change[65]

Sometimes fear of change helps to keep us from successfully shape shifting into our desired form. Diets get boring because we think we have to eat the same bland foods and they get dull. So instead of changing our habits and making an effort, finding a whole new group of foods and seasonings, we lapse back into what's comfortable, known and easy. Overweight is one symptom of this fear. Look at your habits to find out where else you express this fear. No matter how stable or wise we are, change brings out the fragile points of our nature.

Being slender and healthy is definitely going to change your life. People will look at and react to you differently. If you feel that you aren't prepared to handle that, or that you'll resent their sudden acceptance, you're going to avoid that change. Working on that fear from the inside will create positive changes on the outside.

One thing we're afraid of is that life is going to ask of us something that we can't or won't deliver. We believe that there is only enough happiness for a few people and the rest of us have to scramble to get a piece of it. We've forgotten that the Essence doesn't work that way—it will supply us with that upon which we focus. It doesn't take "happy" into consideration; it just gives us what we think about.

Many of us don't think that change can be positive. It's something forced upon us. Even if we are the one making changes, we feel like we're only doing it because something wasn't going right. If someone else would fix things, damn it, then we wouldn't have to! For people who feel this way, change is a victimization process where something is wrong.

---

[65] This section was adapted from a class taught by Victoria Wilson MS, CCE, CHt and an article written by Lisa Bonnice and Victoria Wilson about that same class.

When life changes suddenly we're thrown off track into a new reality, which makes us feel overwhelmed. Some people even get sick when going through change because with such high levels of anxiety, getting sick is the gentlest way of getting through change. They're too sick to give a damn and they won't fight it. If they were completely well and conscious they would have one anxiety attack after another. The illness isn't a punishment - it's actually a more gentle approach to change than we take ourselves through. The shortest distance between two mindsets might be *through* illness!

> Some people get sick when going through change because with such high levels of anxiety, getting sick is the gentlest way of getting through change.

It helps when you realize that change is an unavoidable part of life, because it's the only game in town. *If we didn't change we'd die. Period.* Change is occurring at every moment of every day of every week of every month, etc., ad nauseam. Our energy is moving its positioning and our cells are rebuilding themselves. Nothing stays the same or it dies and decays. Even decaying is a process of change!

Change is why we're here. It's our reason for being. Why would we incarnate if only to stay exactly the same? What's the point? So what are we afraid of? It's like being afraid to breathe! The process of breathing cleans our lungs and renews our oxygen supply for our bodies. It keeps us healthy and alive. So does change. If we're in an unhealthy situation or condition, then we need to breathe new life into it and change it. By focusing on healthy change, making steps in a healthy direction, the change can't help but come out for the better, because that's what we're asking the Essence to deliver!

The whole point of change, of *life*, is to let it alter who we are. Instead of resisting change, we need to say, "This aspect of myself is changing because it can't adequately express the fullness of who I am." Can a child's body adequately express an adolescent? Can an adolescent's body adequately express an adult? Can an unhealthy body adequately express the beauty of our soul? Change *has* to happen. It's the death of what was so that a new level of fullness can come forward.

Self Loathing

Someone says to you, "You look beautiful today!" What is the first thing you do? You point out ALL of your flaws. You feel this oppressive need to prove that person wrong. What if this person had said they love a painting? Would you attack their opinion? What could possibly make you feel so strongly that you act like such a cretin? What are you projecting onto them?

Here's an idea . . . how about taking their word for it?

Do you know how hard it is to give a compliment? Don't you feel like you've just wasted your time when someone denies one that you've offered? Don't you feel like you want to just shake that person or else decide not to bother next time? Do you usually give compliments that you don't mean? If so, are you afraid that others are doing the same to you?

When someone tells you something nice about yourself, pay attention to the things you say to negate them. If these are things you don't like about yourself and for some reason feel the need to point them out, why don't you change these things? They cause you to hate yourself! Make them go away! No need to fear the change, right?

Nocturnal Heebie Jeebies

You know 'em, you love 'em, the Nocturnal Heebie Jeebies (NHJ's[66]) love to wake and keep you up at night, gnawing at your brain. Not only will they keep you awake, they'll jab you with every nagging fear and insecurity you've

[66] You don't really think I'm going to type that out every single time I need to use the phrase do you?

ever had. In fact, when they're on a roll, they'll throw a new one in on ya just for fun.

In an effort to not let them win, I've devised a plan. I've decided to use their methods against them in a Kung Fu kind of way. They say things like "You know that twinge in your gut is cancer, don't you?" and "Your kids hate you. But you knew that, right?" or the infamous, "Christ, you're fat!"[67] I listen to what they say to me and I choose to see their insults as a gift.[68]

By changing my perspective I receive—instead of a sound trouncing from the NHJ's—pure, raw, unfiltered information. These are the background thoughts that are going through my head all day long, sabotaging my shape shifting efforts, but I don't notice them because I'm distracted by traffic, or work, or the thousand other piddly little things that happen throughout the day.

Now that I know what these insidious thoughts are, I can directly counter them with their opposites. In place of fear, I use love. As soon as I recognize that the nighttime wakefulness has shifted into the NHJ's playing field, I begin. I chant an endless string of loving thoughts,[69] like "I am pure love energy." "I am completely healthy—that voice is nothing but fear." "I am the embodiment of forgiveness, both of myself and others." And if that's not working, I resort to the old standby, "I am love, I am love, I am love…"

It takes some doing at first, especially if the NHJ's have formed teams and compete to see who can freak you out the most. What they don't want you to know is that they have no weapons or tools against yours. They can't win as long as you aren't allowing them to stomp you.

---

[67] Let's not even go into the fact that by saying this, one of the most powerful words known to humankind is combined with a heartfelt, self-loathing statement. Just imagine the wallop it packs!

[68] The NHJ's hate that.

[69] Even if I don't believe them. At this point, it doesn't matter. Just do it and you'll be amazed at the results.

It also helps to get up and write them down, promising yourself that you will read them over and take care of the concerns in the light of day. This takes away their power, and then maybe you can sleep.

The best part of this victory is that the process soon becomes second nature, and then begins to filter into your waking life. You'll begin hearing their Heebie Jeebie voices when they pop in during the day, and you can immediately counter them with a *healthy* knee-jerk reaction. You will have kicked some Heebie Jeebie butt.

Doubt

Sometimes our biggest enemy is doubt. You may have even had them while reading this book! New ideas are almost always accompanied by doubt. "This won't work. This is a crock. Yeah, right. This will work for others, maybe, but not me. I can't do that, I'd feel stupid!"

This is important: Doubt is not just fear of failure; it's the ***cause*** of failure. Remember that your words *create your life*. Any doubtful words will create *exactly* what you speak. So if you doubt something is possible, you've just made it impossible with your words! Then your doubts are confirmed!

When we're feeling fear, once again, we're listening to the ego. Doubt can easily slide in when we're manifesting something big, like shape shifting, because one rarely gets *instant* results, so it's incredibly easy to listen to and believe the ego when it pooh-poohs our efforts. "Pooh," it says. "Pooh on that."

Getting past doubt

Before I started working on weight loss, I was desperately trying to work on abundance. It seemed that no matter what I did, I was dirt poor. Sure, I might have had a roof over my head, a car that ran and a job, but I was ultimately poverty-stricken. I owed money to everyone. And I don't mean credit cards or car loans; I didn't have enough money to qualify for credit! The utilities were always a day away from being turned off (sometimes they did get shut off and for long stretches of time). The kids went without insurance and I wore the same clothes for years. I've probably just described some of you.

So, knowing what I do about metaphysics, I followed the rules, which are basically the same as I've laid out for weight loss. Thoughts are things: see yourself wealthy, feel yourself wealthy and you

> ### *This is important:* Doubt is not just fear of failure; it's the *cause* of failure.

will be, blah blah blah. The problem was that it never worked! It took years for me to finally pull out of the poverty mindset because I had so many doubts about my abilities to provide for myself.

It can be incredibly hard to follow metaphysical rules regarding abundance, in real life, when you can't even call the electric company to make payment arrangements because the phone's been cut off! Just struggling to get by took up all my energy. But ironically, I was getting exactly what I was metaphysically asking for. I focused all my energy on how poor I was, and that's what I got.

I think that the *aha!* light bulb finally came on when I read Wayne Dyer's book, *Your Sacred Self* and saw this passage:

". . . if you would really love to manifest prosperity and abundance, but you have doubts about your ability to do so, then first get the visualization of yourself having abundance."

"Then go beyond the picture or image and ask yourself, 'How would I feel if I were to experience this prosperity I visualize?' You would probably think you'd be something like content, fulfilled, grateful, happy or euphoric. These are expressions of feelings that you can generate completely with your inner thoughts.

"Once you can get to the feelings behind your desires and know that you have the capacity to create these feelings by your faith and the discipline of your thoughts, you will realize that needing anything else to feel prosperous is only a belief and is inauthentic. Do this exercise with

anything you wish to create in your life. Go first to the visualization, then to the resultant feeling. Then work at generating that feeling and you will feel your doubts dissipating.[70]

If you didn't get hit with the same lightning bolt as I did, let me spell out what this meant to me. All those years of listening to and reading the same advice, over and over and over, finally sunk in.

All metaphysical books on abundance that I've read say the same thing—in essence, you must *feel* wealthy before you can *be* wealthy. "Uh huh," says I, with the disconnect notice in my hand. But . . . if I am able to feel even *temporary* prosperity in my daydreams—if I can fantasize for *one moment* that I do have unlimited wealth—then the trappings of it are only *solid symbols* of that feeling, because **I was able to create that feeling** of massive wealth and it was just as real as anything solid you see before you.

To be sure, this brief moment of prosperous thinking will not help me pay that bill by itself. However, if I build up enough of those moments, like atoms of identical structure, eventually they will create the physical substance of that moment, which is abundance in my life.

Understand? I really don't need the *stuff* to be able to feel wealth. I've just felt wealth! That's all I really wanted the *stuff* for anyway, to feel the freedom from stress that wealth brings.

I know the question remains, what about the bills? Don't let that question shatter your new blissful moments . . . instead, look at them as fallout—leftovers—from your past thoughts that needs to be taken care of. Your new thoughts aren't going to make bills disappear, because they're already physical—a karmic result of past actions. However, your new thoughts may help to attract some extra cash out of the blue!

If I can feel wealth without the stuff, who really needs it!? By being in those feelings more and more often, you further

---

[70] *Your Sacred Self,* Wayne Dyer, Harper Mass Market Paperbacks; (March 1996) ISBN: 0061094757

114

energize your wealthy feeling. Eventually stuff will just start to show up in your life because it's what you're attracting with the wealth vibe.

This is what it means when they say, "you must feel wealthy to be wealthy," or "it takes money to make money." This same advice can be used for any shape shifting goal. In order to be thinner, we have to be able to *feel* what it would be like to be thin.

How would it make you feel to be in the body you desire? Sexier? Lighter? Prettier? Faster? Healthier? Make a list of words and then place yourself within the feelings that they bring up. Connect to those feelings in your mind and feel them in your body. Attach yourself to those feelings and you will *be* thin in that moment. Don't look in the mirror and say things like, "Yeah, right!" You will be thinner every day, once you begin to attach to the feelings.

For example, if I were thinner, I'd buy new clothes, because I didn't want to spend money on fat clothes. I always thought I'd lose weight and those big clothes would be a waste of money.

However, if being thinner to me means looking better, and if I buy just a couple new outfits, then I'll look better. That's what I was shooting for to begin with!

If I was thinner, I'd feel sexier. But since I'm not, I'll just slump around with bad posture and talk about how ugly I am so others will know that I know and they don't have to tell me.

On the other hand, if being thinner means feeling sexier, I can do that without too much problem. There are other things that can make you feel sexual, whether it's lingerie, candles, woman-friendly porn … whatever. It's all in your mind and you can use external tools to help you to get into that mindset. You don't need the shape shift to feel sexual! But you do need the sexual in order to shape shift—sexual energy is creative energy and without it, you're just treading water.

Once we stop focusing so strongly on the body we hate, and start treating it as though it were attractive, then your shape can naturally start to shift (provided we aren't sabotaging ourselves in some other way).

Another great trick along these lines is that you can carry that feeling thing a step further. For example, just a few minutes ago, I was just sort of daydreaming, and I started thinking how much I'd love an ice cream bar. I have them in the freezer, and I would like to have one right now. However, I really didn't feel like getting up to get it. So I just sort of imagined what it would be like to have one.

Once you stop focusing so strongly on the body you hate, and start treating it as though it were attractive, then your shape can naturally start to shift.

Then I realized that I really didn't want that. It would make me feel kind of sluggish and heavy, so I wondered what else I had in the kitchen.

I remembered that I had just bought a can of gingered pears and that sounded even better! Not only that, but it was a classier dessert than just a dumb old ice cream bar—the kind of thing you might get in a restaurant.

So my mind wandered to Paris, where I was eating gingered pears in a little sidewalk café. In fact, there was ice cream in the bowl, with the pears on top and the syrup from the pears was thinning the ice cream, just a touch.

I could feel how cold my teeth were when I took a bite, and could taste the blend of the pears with the cool, melted vanilla ice cream. It suddenly dawned on me; this is what I've been talking about! I just had an incredible dessert—in Paris, of all places! I was there! I lived it! I didn't even need the real thing now, because I just had the feeling of being there! And that's all I really wanted anyway—the feeling that my daydream had just given me.

116

Now if you were able to come with me as I described it, then you were there, too! You don't need the ice cream either.

Isn't the mind an amazing thing?

Why does it have to be so hard?

Losing weight can be one of the hardest things you'll ever do, especially when the attitude of many people is that it's a snap and *you* must just be weak if you can't do it.

Think of it this way. You've put on the weight for a reason. This is the way you have chosen to bury your issues. Some people find other ways, like drugs, or obsessions, etc. That's another reason they are thin and we aren't.[71] Instead of resolving an issue or reacting to it in another unhealthy way, we buried it in excess flesh. In order to take it back off, we must resolve that issue. And this can hurt. Your ego has a field day keeping you from this pain.

You've allowed that pain energy to solidify by suppressing or hanging onto feelings, instead of letting the energy of anger, pain, resentment, etc., flow through you as it's first happening.

Once you loosen the energy around an issue, as you will whenever you go through any personal growth, it's going to come up. You may not end up reliving specific incidents or experience, but the pain of it might start to surface physically, like a zit. You'll get a chest pain, or some sort of symptoms and your ego will say, "Alert! Alert! You're dying! Look over here!" and the issue gets buried right back where it was. Hence, the solid energy, the fat, won't go away.

In my opinion, a hypochondriac is just someone who is sensitive to his/her own energy body, but is either unaware that it exists or of how to fix it. He/she knows there's something wrong, but the doctor can't find any physical sign of it **yet**. The feeling of illness in your body begins on the energy level. You're aware that something doesn't feel right.

[71] Unless they have drug *and* weight problems!

You have a little twinge here or pain there, or a tingle or whatever physical twitch that occurs.

The feeling continues because the energy field in that area of the body is disturbed. If you don't know how to repair or smooth that area, especially if you are completely unaware of how energy works, and the stressors that are causing the disturbance continue, the disturbed energy will continue to grow until it begins to solidify as your body. It's like when you feel a pimple growing. It's sort of itchy and tingly, but there is no sign yet of physical disturbance. You, however, know that something is amiss.

Once symptoms become more solidified and frightening, you finally go to the doctor because it feels like a "legitimate" illness. It's still not solid enough for a doctor to see there is something wrong. So you're sent home with a pat on the head and a bill in your hand. You go home and **worry worry worry**, because *you* know there's something amiss, thereby focusing your energy on it even further. This helps to gel and solidify that energy. Eventually you will have worked yourself into an actual physical dis-ease. You will have shifted your shape into one that includes illness. But at least you'll have the satisfaction of saying "I told you so!"

The feeling of illness in your body begins on the energy level in your aura if you aren't living your truth—resonating with the Essence. Depending on what level of the aura is disturbed and the corresponding chakra, the physical twinges will be in a specific part of the body.

So, for example, if you're not seeing your self clearly or are refusing to look at something that needs to be examined, your eyes may begin to get weak.

If you need to speak up about something, and stand your ground, or if you're not speaking the truth, the fifth chakra will become disturbed energetically. As long as this continues, the energy may begin to solidify and manifest as a sore throat, or some other illness in the throat area.

For example: I was meditating recently, when I wasn't feeling very well. I had been fighting a horrible cold and had

118

developed bronchitis. I was coughing and hacking, I had a sore throat and wasn't getting much sleep. One morning I woke up with chest pains—not emergency room type pains, but goopy lung pains. Anyway, as I was lying there meditating I was wondering why I was so sick and made a mental note to look up my symptoms in my mind/body reference book when I got up (*The Body Mind Workbook* by Debbie Shapiro[72] . . . an *amazing* book).

As I was lying there, my chest started hurting again and my throat was burning. I thought about the chakras in those locations and realized that the chest pain (heart chakra) meant I wasn't allowing myself enough love energy and my throat hurt because I wasn't communicating something, but I didn't know what. So I focused on my heart chakra and visualized streams of love energy filling my body, through that chakra.

My chest pains got stronger and I heard my ego telling me I was going to die if I kept this up. I actually began wondering if I should go to the emergency room. I remembered seeing Wayne Dyer on TV recently, talking about his heart attack (synchronicity, anyone?). He said that as he was in the ER, really scared, he asked God for help. He said, "I don't know how to do this. Help me."

So I opened to Spirit and asked for help. I said, "I don't know what's going on here. This really hurts and I'm getting scared. What should I do?" My intuition told me to just breathe through it and let it come. Follow my own advice that I've been writing here.

That's what I did. I took deep breaths and saw the energy pouring into me. I felt a lot of pain and was afraid that I was fooling myself—that I was going to die right there. As I continued with the energy, I felt stronger and stronger and realized that even if I did die, it would only be my body. *I would continue.*

The pain started dissipating and spreading out. I suddenly thought of an instance where my feelings were very deeply

---

[72] *The Body Mind Workbook;* Debbie Shapiro; Element Books; 1990

hurt by something someone said about my body. I felt the pain of that moment again, but continued to breathe through it. The moment passed and the pain was gone, almost instantly.[73]

After I felt better, I did look up the symptoms to see what it was that I was ignoring or fighting. Interestingly enough, a cold is ". . . often synonymous with needing time out to reconnect with our inner selves and with our desire to live; it is a way of releasing pent-up frustration or emotions to do with inner change." [74]

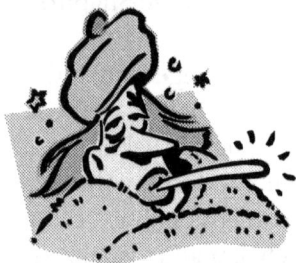

It also says, "Catching a cold usually occurs when we need time out from what we are doing, when there are emotional issues bothering us that need to be released or when the relationship between our mind and body is not in harmony. A cold reminds us of crying; the same watery eyes and wet nose, the same sniffing and sense of despair, the same need to be loved yet also to be alone. Is there something we would really like to be crying about but are not admitting?" [75]

After I typed those last few paragraphs I became too sick to write for a while. I went from a cold, to a sinus infection, then straight into pneumonia—at the tail end of the pneumonia my period started, complete with huge clots and deluging flow. All I could really do was lie around feeling

---

[73] Medical disclaimer: just because I did this, doesn't mean you should ignore serious medical symptoms. Please don't ignore a real heart problem because I worked through this. If you feel it's serious, then go ahead and get help, AND breathe through it. By the way, once the pain of the memory was over, I could not remember what the original insult was, no matter how hard I tried!

[74] *The Body Mind Workbook;* Debbie Shapiro; Element Books; 1990; p122

[75] Ibid

120

awful. From time to time I'd try to sit at the computer, but just couldn't make myself even open this document.

I then figured that if that wasn't going to work, I'd at least make sure I journaled, because I could lie down and do that. Nope, didn't do that either. So I'll read. I'll do some research on the topic so I can maybe get back into it. Nada.

Nothing I tried helped me to get any further work done on this book. In addition, I gained back every inch that I had previously lost (three inches in the hips and two in the waist).

Something must have been seriously bothering me, or my body wouldn't be fighting my mind so hard like that. To become so sick that I become entirely ineffective and so thoroughly sidetracked, there must have been some deep issues that my ego didn't want me dredging up. I'd been working so hard, and concentrating so much on this book, that I was bringing up a lot of information and working through a lot of stuff.

Back to the mind/body connection: the cold, as it says above, "reminds us of crying; the same watery eyes and wet nose, the same sniffing and sense of despair, the same need to be loved yet also to be alone. Is there something we would really like to be crying about but are not admitting?"[76]

I spent a huge portion of that time while I was sick just bawling my eyes out. I would just start sobbing, for no real reason. This was before even looking up the cause and effect of colds.

However, if I let myself really feel why I was crying so hard, I would always come up with something. I hated my job. Therefore, I hated my life. I felt used and neglected and unappreciated. I resented having to work there just for the money when there were things I needed to be doing—would *rather* be doing, instead. My calling was elsewhere, but I was viciously stuck in a place I didn't want to be.

Add feelings of guilt and being an ingrate to this, because it really was a pretty good job and I should have been grateful

[76] Ibid

that I had it. It offered me tremendous opportunities and invaluable experience. Plus, what makes me any different from anyone else who hates his or her job or doesn't want to work?[77] What makes me so special that I should be able to not work, when everyone else has to? At least being sick I didn't have to be there. I could take a few sick days.

Since a cold won't keep you out of the office for too long, and I hadn't done anything to change my circumstances, the illness progressed into something more serious, a sinus infection and a couple more missed days at work. I didn't have the confidence that I could find another job that I'd like more and ended up having to suffer with this illness as a result. *It wasn't a conscious choice* to get sick. I only realized this in hindsight, and it proved to me how powerful the subconscious is.

With that sinus infection, a doctor gave me a narcotic cough medicine, which gave me such horribly vivid dreams that I was afraid to sleep. The basic theme of all the dreams was that part of me wanted to change for the better but was afraid of what would happen if I did. For example, in one dream I was in the mall trying on new clothes, clothes that would fit my newly thin body, and I was having a great time. I went into the fitting room and there was a murderer in there, waiting to kill me. All the other dreams, although different story lines, told the same tale.

So now if we look up sinus infection, it says, "The sinuses are the air passages in our head and are related to your more abstract and thinking processes, to awareness and to communication. An inflammation also suggests an emotional anger or irritation; the discharge is also emotional (fluid), a release of negative emotions or a state of being emotionally overwrought. Sinusitis can therefore indicate a deep conflict

---

[77] A huge segment of society!

122

or release of negativity in the area of abstract activity, of thinking, and in our communication." [78]

I think that sort of speaks for itself, but since you're not inside my mind, I'll elaborate. I've already made it plain that I hated my job and was desperate to not work there, but I didn't do anything to change it. I was afraid to get another job because what if things were even worse there? What if it turns out that the job I'd had was a piece of cake compared to some other job that I'd hate even more? Therein lies the emotional anger part.

Abstract thinking processes and communication were absolutely necessary to what I was trying to write in this book. Again, some fear was keeping me from digging into abstract thoughts and communicating them. A sinus infection was certainly keeping me from doing any of that. I felt like I had completely lost touch with my spiritual side. I felt totally lost and alone, and when I would ask Universal Intelligence for help, I didn't feel any connection.

Now let's take a look at pneumonia. According to the author, "The lungs are where we take in breath, which is life; without it we die. The lungs are our means for separate life, for here we breathe alone. However, there are times when breathing is not so much fun—maybe when life has become somewhat overwhelming, or there is conflict within us about living our lives for ourselves versus being in a very close or dominating relationship. Then our ability to breathe may become diminished, or we may feel stifled. An inflammation indicates that this area has become hot and angry, irritated or frustrated. It is red and sore and it makes breathing very difficult. So our desire and ability to breathe have become severely affected by our emotion; by our fears of being alone or of being overwhelmed; by our anger towards life or

[78] *The Body Mind Workbook;* Debbie Shapiro; Element Books; 1990; p163

towards our aloneness and to actually being here, or by our irritation with ourselves." [79]

Heavy stuff. Let's look at it again. I said earlier, "I resent having to work there just for the money when there are things I need to be doing instead." You know what the voice in my head said as soon as I typed that? It said, "Oh, you and about a million other people."

I'm willing to bet that you thought that as well, something along the lines of, "Poor baby. Join the club." But that's not the way it's got to be! One reason to be stuck in a job you hate is fear; another is because of the attachment to the hate. It reproduces itself because that's what you're focusing on.

Now I had to look at what I feared, what kept me stuck in a life that made me so miserable. It must be something pretty huge, if it could keep me literally trapped in a day-to-day existence that I found so loathsome that I gave myself pneumonia as a *happier* alternative!!! Here's where journaling can come in handy, if you can force yourself to do it!

Here is some stream of consciousness writing that I put in my journal while I was sick and trying to figure out why I couldn't get better or write anything.

> *I want to quit my job so badly that I cry about it all the time. I make myself sick so I don't have to go to work. But I don't want to find another job. I don't want another job. I want to stay home and write.*
>
> *I keep getting fatter and fatter, and the book I'm trying to write is supposed to be about weight loss. I can't write cuz I'm so sick and I feel like I've lost my connection to spirit.*
>
> *Sometimes I feel like I can't really make any of this metaphysical stuff work, because I just don't get it. I think I have a grasp of a concept, but it doesn't work. I feel like everyone else gets it, but I don't.*

[79] *The Body Mind Workbook;* Debbie Shapiro; Element Books; 1990; p158

What is the benefit of holding on to the belief that I'm the only one who can't connect?

Because if I can connect, I'd be responsible for my own life. If I'm responsible for my own life, I have no one to blame when it goes wrong. I have no one to depend on to catch me when I fall. I'll have to do it all myself.

What am I afraid will happen if I change?

The me that is will die.

I had already decided long ago that I want to be responsible for my own life now, so the belief that I can't connect is obsolete—it isn't a benefit anymore. I just hung on to it out of habit. Turns out that whatever I was afraid of is really not very scary at all, but look how hard I fought to not see it! Rather, look how hard my ego fought to keep itself alive: "**the me that is will die.**"

Please pardon what appears to be indulgence while I continue to talk about something that doesn't look at all related to weight loss, but that's the point I'm trying to make. It's not the food. It's the garbage in our lives that we avoid— the stuff we won't let go of—that becomes physical fat, that shifts our shape!

Here's the cool, happy ending. After a month of being very ill, and finally working through the above, I began to feel a lot better. (I was a little annoyed that I gained those inches back.)

My financial situation started changing and I was able to eventually quit my job. It wasn't that I didn't want to work; I just didn't want to work *there.* I wanted to work out of my home, making/selling jewelry and writing.

I knew I could do it, but I was terrified to take the leap of faith that I would be okay without a regular weekly paycheck and insurance.

Another truly frightening thing was writing this book, something I've never done before. I've got *years* of professional writing experience, but not on my own book! In addition, it's on a real hot issue, something that millions of people have a problem with. I'm trying to prove that my method is worth writing a book about, so I had bloody well be losing weight successfully doing this! This has to work! I'm trying very hard to be accurate and not to be misleading, because I'm not a snake-oil salesman, and I have nightmares about people calling me a charlatan (projecting my own fears that I don't know what the hell I'm talking about onto my work). This fear is pretty disabling—enough to keep me too sick to sit at the keyboard, don't you think? After all, if I'm too sick to write, then I never have to face that fear!

Here's a metaphor that keeps appearing to me when I think of a visual for the way that month of illness looked. It's almost as if a huge chunk of land with a house on it is being wiggled out of the middle of a jigsaw puzzle of earth . . . like an unseen crane is lifting this square plot of land, with a lot of earthquake type activity and gnashing of teeth. Once the plot of land was lifted free of the earth, it was turned 90 degrees and plopped back down into the square hole. Now everything has settled down to earth, but is facing another direction. Life is basically the same—same house, same area, just a new direction. Changing to this direction was very unsettling and difficult, but now the change has been made and my illness kept me from getting in my own way.

One more brief illustration of the body/mind connection is that I've spent the majority of my lifetime denying my femininity. It was even difficult for me to actually type the phrase "my femininity" just because I didn't want to own it. "I didn't ask for it, don't say it's mine!" I hated being female so much that I sent *huge* amounts of hatred and loathing energy toward my physical expression of being female, my reproductive system. So much so that I manifested horrible periods, with (turn your eyes if you're squeamish) blood clots as big as a bar of soap, blood simply *pouring* out of me, cramps that cripple and weakness that kept me in bed for days.

I had seen countless doctors about it and they couldn't find anything "wrong," so it must "just be the way I am." I had to live with it. This is why we develop serious illness, because it can't be "cured" until it's a "disease!" Sometimes, until we unearth the cause of illness, it can't be cured. In the same way, some of us can't lose weight until we figure out why we gained it!

The power of the thoughts of others

Obesity in this country is being called an epidemic. Studies have shown that in the past few decades, Americans have become heavier and heavier. It's an alarming trend that the medical world is studying but they haven't come up with any solid "whys." They blame fast food, lack of exercise, etc., but they don't know why changing diet and exercise doesn't work for everyone.

The Journal of the American Medical Association (JAMA) says that between 1991 and 1998, the percentage of the population defined as dangerously overweight was up almost 50%.[80] However, they don't mention any corollary between this epidemic and the beginning of media pressure to be ultra thin.

Naomi Wolf wrote, in her classic book *The Beauty Myth*, "During the past decade,[81] women breached the power structure; meanwhile, eating disorders rose exponentially and cosmetic surgery became the fastest-growing medical specialty. During the past five years, consumer spending doubled, pornography became the main media category, ahead of legitimate films and records combined, and 33,000 American women told researchers that they would rather lose ten to fifteen pounds than achieve any other goal."[82]

---

[80] The Spread of the Obesity Epidemic in the United States, 1991-1998 Ali H. Mokdad; Mary K. Serdula; William H. Dietz; Barbara A. Bowman; James S. Marks; Jeffrey P. Koplan; JAMA.999;282:1519-1522
[81] She's talking about the 1980's
[82] The Beauty Myth; Naomi Wolf; Harperperennial Library; ISBN: 0060512180; (September 24, 2002)

In these same past few decades, as we as a culture have been getting heavier, the pressure has been extraordinarily heavy from external sources to look a certain way. In centuries past, there have been styles and body shapes in vogue, but those populations weren't inundated in their daily lives with images that they are supposed to live up to.

The sheer *volume* of messages that we receive is overwhelmingly greater than ever before in our history. The energetic power of the message that we're not good enough is more than we can metabolize, especially if we're not even aware that it's working us.

To reiterate, we are being spoon-fed the message that we are not as good as we can be because we don't look like "that." And we gobble it up as fast as they can shovel it in. This isn't necessarily a deliberate, evil, mean thing that anyone is doing to hurt us. They're simply making money. Caveat emptor. Chances are good that they actually believe their own garbage. Forgive them Father, they know not what they do.

> **The energetic power of the message that we're not good enough is more than we can metabolize, especially if we're not even aware that it's working us.**

However, look at the difference between, for example, a stadium with one light bulb shining in the middle of the floor, and that same stadium with a light bulb lit in every single seat. The difference in energy flow between these two is astronomical. That's the volumes of energy behind this relatively new message that we are receiving.

People who can cash in on it are pushing the message, "You are too fat," onto us in order to sell their products, and it's reinforced by us when we buy into it. *You are too fat*—the energy push is just overwhelming. *You are too fat*—the message comes from all sides. *You are too fat*—if your energy isn't strong enough to fight it (*you are too fat*), you don't stand a chance. The power and strength of this energetic force is actually causing us to be heavy, if we do not have our self-esteem shield in place!

By working through the issues that allow our energy to be sapped and our self-esteem destroyed, we can begin to build up our strength to fight those false messages.

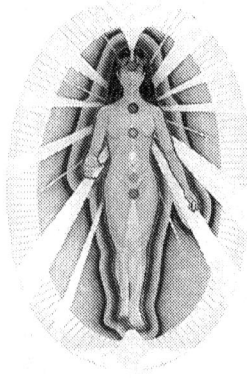

SHIFTING YOUR SHAPE

Think yourself thin

Let's review just a little bit:

A solid has a slower rate of vibration than a liquid or gas of the same substance. Its shape and density is determined by the elements contained within.

Each element—the building blocks of physicality like carbon, iron, and oxygen—has its own unique vibration. Each vibration has its own "Is" that is uniquely it.

That vibration is what tells an element's atoms what shape to form and vice versa. The tiniest change in vibration changes it from one element to the other. Hydrogen vibrates at one, the tone or sound that one electron would make. Add another electron and you have a slightly different tone—it becomes helium. Add another and you'll have lithium, etc.

Different combinations of the elements' metaphysical properties result in different things, which all *feel* different. So our unique combination of the elements' properties and their corresponding emotions are what makes a solid "us."

A solid item has its own vibrational makeup. This explains how crystals work in healing us. Like a tuning fork, they hold a similar

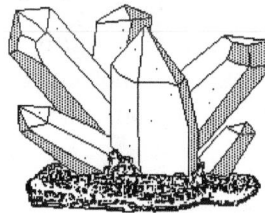

vibration as a healthy heart, liver, kidney, etc., just as a healthy chakra will have healthy organs associated with it. Having the crystal close will align that part of us with the healthy vibe, almost like a teacher—it shows the organ how to be.

The energy that is "us" is simply a solidification of various elements, which correspond to our emotions and sensations. Our emotions and sensations are the vibes that shape our bodies.

We might carry a vibe that corresponds to being low in the metaphysical properties of iron, for example. This is how an iron deficiency can create changes in every facet of your being. A facet of our behavior that corresponds to that lack may be something simple like an aversion to veggies like spinach, which has its own properties. That element is in low supply and "X" properties go with it and vice versa. You now vibrate at a different rate than you would if you had enough iron, and your body is going to slowly change its physical shape into a state that doesn't resonate with health, like iron-poor blood.

Our thoughts control the shape we shift into. Through those thoughts—emotions and sensations that we allow to linger—we rearrange those elements into different shapes. There are a *lot* of *strongly* previously trained molecules to shift, so it's not an instantaneous process. It takes time and focused thought to change that shape.

The thought "I am a disgusting pig," resonates with the unhealthy vibration of excess human fat (feelings and visualization along with firm conviction that it's true) that causes a reaction in your body—the creation and accumulation of fat.

To counteract the solidification of that fat vibe, you simply reverse the process, using the same formula: feelings + visualization + firm conviction = electrical, chemical, physical reaction. One way to do that is with affirmations, but they must be done correctly **and with patience** or they're useless.

Affirmations

Affirmations work like a charm for many people but not for others. If they don't work for you, then you must take small steps at first, while you learn how to use them. It's difficult to start out with affirmations that you currently think are lies, like "I am beautiful," because you just plain will not believe it yet. That's why affirmations don't work for so many people. They are empty words that make us feel worthless when we don't see any changes. We have a bridge to cross first. You can't get from Monday to Friday without going through the rest of the week.

For the past 20 years or so, I've dedicated myself to the study of "creating my reality." That was the buzz phrase of countless books that I've read—*How to Create Your Own Reality*. If only I'd known then that there is no "how to." It's more like "just is." "How to" implies *future* results. The secret lies in the **NOW**.

For a very long time I misunderstood these books and my life continued to suck. What I didn't get was *why* my life still sucked while I did affirmations and thought positive and burned incense and cast spells and all the other stuff that goes along with New Age thought.

Affirmations tend to imply what you **want** to be, not what you are. This, in and of itself, is fine, as long as you're not jumping too far ahead of yourself. Start small, with something that you already like about yourself, something that already exists. Find things you like and affirm them.

This will bring those aspects of yourself to the forefront and give them a chance to be displayed more often. In turn, this will help you to dig deeper and find other things that you are happy with. In this way you pull good things out of yourself that *already exist*, not just things with the potential to exist. Those potential things may only come about after you've acknowledged and affirmed what you already are.

Affirmations are just thoughts—energy, steered by our emotions and reactions to circumstances. That flow, since it is active, causes a reaction when it blends with passive energy, the energy of our auric field.

In other words, thought is the artist's hands in the clay of Essence. When we think, we are directing our energy into the pliable Essence energy. This is how we create our reality.

Everything we think, and I do mean *every single thing*,[83] causes the Essence to ripple, in order to form a solid version of those thoughts. So if our predominant thoughts are about how fat and ugly we are, then we are just going to continue being that. This is why it's so very important to remain upbeat and soul-connected.

> **Thought is the artist's hands in the clay of Essence. When we think, we are directing our energy into the pliable Essence energy.**

The *occasional* affirmation or positive thought isn't enough to overpower the majority of the negative thoughts, especially since we're usually unaware of the loop playing the Heebie Jeebies in the background. The positive ones have to take up at least 51 percent of your thoughts in order to stand a chance. The higher the percentage that you spend on the positive, the more quickly you'll get results. By affirming things that are already true, it's easier to push past the 50% mark.

If an affirmation is true for you now, then you can easily skate through the day repeating this to yourself, probably just as easily as you tell yourself, for example, how disgusting you are. That comes naturally anymore and is the truth for you. Hence, the body that disgusts you. So you start out with something like "I care enough about myself to give this process some thought." You can even try for something personal that you like about yourself, even something as mild

---

[83] It may seem like I'm pounding this into the ground, but it is essential that you remember this.

as "I'm kind to animals." Find the things about yourself that you really do like and pat yourself on the back for them.

These easy thoughts are the first steps across the bridge to an "I am beautiful" reality. They demonstrate that you are deserving of and actively living "love."

The next step goes a little further, with something that you wouldn't have believed yesterday, but you can believe today. Every day, dig up more stuff about yourself that you like, because you'll be able to now that you've started the process.

One of the most powerful affirmations I've ever used was one that I didn't even realize was an affirmation. Bear with me while I share a brief bit of background first.

All my life I've always felt like there was a gray cloud over me, blocking the sun. Everyone else seemed happy, or at least content, but I always had this melancholia that kept me from connecting to them and their happiness. Basically, I was chronically depressed. Nothing ever really worked for me, even though I have a lot of various abilities and was good at using them. I just never really succeeded at anything because I had a major fear of success—like I didn't deserve it.

However, once in a while, every couple weeks or so, I would get a flash of a moment of clarity, a brief, powerful second of feeling totally alive and connected and understanding what life is supposed to feel like. Sometimes it would occur when I heard an old song that I loved, or smelled fall leaves, and sometimes with no stimuli. It was like a mini orgasm, just out of the blue, and it was heartbreaking when it faded away, elusive as the gossamer memory of a dream as you wake up.

In the meantime, a similar pattern would play out in my life. I'd be pretty happy for a day or two, sometimes a week, and feel like I really had it all together. But then, out of the blue, I'd be dashed back into feeling like there was really no reason to get out of bed.

I talked to my spiritual teacher[84] about this, wondering what it was and why I was being tortured with the knowledge of something that I couldn't seem to have. She suggested that I look at my life as having a brick wall built around me, and these flashes were like holes in the wall that I could see through to the other side. On that other side is the way life is supposed to feel when we're soul connected. That's what I was feeling—brief moments of soul connection.

Then she suggested that when I get one of these flashes, I should try to make the hole in the wall just a little larger and make that feeling last a little longer. She said that this other side of the wall is what we're supposed to feel, that it's a realistic goal—it's what we're all shooting for.

Knowing that I really could have this, that "deserve" had nothing to do with it, helped me to focus on expanding those moments of bliss. They began lasting a little longer and coming more frequently. The more I enjoyed them, the more they enjoyed coming. It was like meeting an old friend, one who really had my best interest at heart. Eventually, the holes in the wall got big enough for me to look through regularly. If I felt down, I just looked through one of the holes and worked on making it bigger.

At the moment of this writing, I feel like the wall has been reduced to piles of bricks. There is still a lot of clearing away to do of the rubbish that the wall was made from, but at least I can see beyond them now. And I can smell the air and live in the vibe of the reality that was only outside the wall before. If/when I get depressed now, it doesn't last more than a couple days and the periods of feeling pretty darned good can last for a month or two, sometimes longer, if I'm really on a roll. I've learned to recognize when I'm staring at the pile of bricks instead of the light. And the best thing is, I know that it only gets better from here, as long as I keep focusing on the bliss instead of the pile of trash.

[84] Victoria Wilson MS, CCE, CHt

This may not appear, on the surface, to have much to do with affirmations. But it beautifully illustrates the process. What I didn't realize at the time was that my focusing on those moments of light was an affirmation that this is how life could be. Every time I focused my thoughts on this ecstasy it became a little more real. I was affirming, without words, what would become. If I'd started by affirming that I could feel bliss all the time, but had still never experienced it, I would have no basis for comparison—nothing to anchor my focus on—so I couldn't have made it real. I would simply be affirming that there is something that I'm *trying* to feel but can't. Therefore, what would become my reality is that **there is something that I'm trying to feel but can't**.

So what affirmations can we use for shape shifting into weight loss? Make them up as you go along. Next time you pass up a candy bar, pat yourself on the back and make that an affirmation. "I can easily pass up a candy bar." When you've noticed that you're beginning to feel better after changing your eating habits to be healthier, affirm, "I feel better every day and this new way of eating is truly worthwhile." If you "fall off the wagon" after a period of doing really well, affirm, "I was able to live for (how many) days without blowing it. I can easily do it again, and I can start right now."[85]

Affirmations can be very powerful if used correctly. Just remember that an affirmation that feels like a lie may not work. Find a lesser version of what you wish to be true and work up to it, adding onto it every chance you get. This is how we create our reality, by actually *making* it happen, by *being* the change. Too many people think that metaphysics, and therefore shape shifting, means something mystical and

---

[85] Don't wait until tomorrow to get back on the horse. If you blew it at lunch, accept it and live the rest of the day as though you hadn't. If you did it at dinner, don't figure that you can just go ahead and have three pieces of cake because you've already blown it for the night and will begin again tomorrow. We both know that you won't get back on unless you do it right now.

occult, something that only a chosen few can understand. It's not.

You're doing it right now.

You just did it again.

There you go again.

You see? It flows like water in a river. The water erodes rocks in its way and changes their form. Your thoughts, likewise, flow constantly, eroding and reshaping your physical form, whether you are aware of it or not.

It's the basic rules of life, the common sense things that you already know. You must use A+B to make C. You can't have C without A and B. It's difficult to shift into and reclaim your perfect shape unless you go through the equation. Our problem is that we think the equation is either a waste of time, or too painful, or too long to wait, or (insert your favorite excuse here). We don't enjoy the process. We just want the end result. And by *wanting* the end result, we continue to project it into our future.

Working with the Essence

Now that you have a sense of the basics, you can perhaps feel comfortable enough to convincingly work with the Essence. What I mean by this is to send your thoughts deliberately into the energy field in which you float, with the intention of creating physical changes.

The Essence doesn't so much communicate in words as much as it does in a single moment of vibration, because that moment is all that is, at that moment. The Essence lives in the *now*. What you think now is what it starts making *now*. A perfect example is the story I told above about affirmations. I focused on the bliss in the Essence and it expanded, becoming more a part of my life with every time I did so.

Again using the formula above, *feelings + visualization + firm conviction*, combine these elements into one brief moment of realization of what you desire. Work toward imagining what it will feel like for you when your body looks its best. Actually allow yourself to *feel* it, the comfort of well fitting clothes, crossing your legs more easily, wearing a swim suit in public, climbing stairs without losing your breath, not sweating as much—the whole nine yards.

The more strongly you can conjure up these feelings, the more firm your conviction that you can be this way, then in that one moment you actually are that way.

Try to picture what you'll realistically look like then, in a comfortable environment, where you feel loved and relaxed— perhaps trim and healthy and in a close family moment, or on a mountaintop—wherever you need to be to feel your best. Allow these two to drift together until their combination is greater than their sum. The more strongly you can conjure up these feelings, the more firm your conviction that you can be this way, then ***in that one moment you actually are*** that way. Remember it's the feeling that we're looking for, not the physical stuff.

IMPORTANT NOTE: Make sure you add healthy, happy and harming no one into the picture. Otherwise you may end up getting thin but as a result of something not so good, like an illness or from depression over a death of a loved one, or whatever. Remember that ***you will get what you ask for***. If you don't specify how you want it, you'll get it in whatever way the Essence chooses for you. It has no emotion, remember? The Essence doesn't know that you didn't want AIDS as a way to lose weight. It just delivered what you asked for and you may have just asked for "fast weight loss."[86] Sometimes the shortest distance between two states of mind is through illness or trauma.

Another important note is that you should leave other people out of it as much as possible because then their assistance may be necessary to create the changes. If you include someone in your projected bliss who doesn't play along and tries to hold you back, it will take much longer for you to achieve your goal because you'll be dragging them along kicking and screaming. Better to do it *yourself* and more easily.

When I say above that you can use a close family moment, you don't even have to specify which family members, especially if you have an unhealthy family relationship. Just bring up a feeling of being with a loving family, whomever that may include in the future bliss moment. There may be people you haven't even met yet involved in that future picture! Or leave the word "family" out entirely but concentrate on feeling loved. Remember, family isn't always the people we're related to by blood.

Once you've captured that single moment of those things combined, you've touched the vibe, that bliss, that you are working toward. That vibration actually exists now. Ten minutes ago it didn't. You've just created the "thin, happy you" vibe. Even if you have momentarily lost it, and don't feel connected to it right now, this doesn't mean you didn't create it. You just aren't allowing yourself to resonate with it at this specific moment.

You can bring that vibe back at any time, because it's part of you. You created it. It's in your field and has already begun to make ripples. The more often you connect to it, the more you feed it, the more it will harden the Essence until it becomes substantial enough for you to not have to try. As this happens, you'll find that you're slowly gaining health, and just naturally making better choices for yourself.

[86] An extreme example, but it brings the point home.

This new vibration in your field will begin to attract you to healthier foods, simply because they resonate with your new vibe. You might still have a *taste* for gooey pastries and stuff, but you'll find that to eat them doesn't do the job for you anymore because they don't resonate with you. They may just be too darned sweet and you have enough sweetness in your life these days. Maybe it's something rich that you eat. But rich food doesn't fit anymore because your energy field is rich enough. You'll also notice that you're not as hungry anymore because you feel full enough.

The only thing that can cause the process to fail is this: losing patience and letting doubt creep in. *Physical results may not appear overnight.* The second you think, "This isn't working," you'll need to go back a few steps and start from where you think you can jump back in. I bet you don't have to start at the beginning. So at least some progress is made. Chances are you were moving too quickly and weren't resonating yet with the vibe you're shooting for. You don't "get it" yet. You're only on Wednesday, and you think it should be Friday.

> **Once you've captured that single moment, you've touched the vibe, that bliss, that you are working toward. That vibration actually exists now.**

You can do visualizations that help your energy begin to reshape itself, and this will boost and support your other work, synergistically.

Imagine that spark of life that went into the vibe you created. Relive the vibe and build it up as much as you can. Picture it as a spark of light that you're growing within you, like an egg is projected into the uterus, and resting on the endometrium (the Essence). Now you'll have a visual focal point upon which to project your creative energy.

Imagine that spark growing into a new being in the womb. That being is the new you. It is growing with the vibration

141

that you created and projected—a thin, healthy, happy you. If you're picturing it as outside of yourself, then bring that visualization inside. Overlay this image of the womb (yes, even men) with this spark inside in the area of the second chakra where sexual "creative" energy resides, just below your navel. See the image of the new spark of life growing within you, glowing with an intense orange light.

Now, imagine that you really are pregnant—creating a new life (yes, men too.) Treat your body with extra special care because what you bring in also goes to the "baby." Care for your body the same way you would if you were responsible for the life of someone you deeply love.

As you care for and nurture your spark, you'll sense it growing and becoming more a part of you. You can actually now see what your body is beginning to look like, just like you imagined for the creation of the spark. It's getting more and more solid, and bigger and bigger and eventually it becomes a solid enough energy mass that it becomes you. It discards excess energy (fat) that it doesn't need to be what it is.

That discarded energy is leftover emotions, traumas, anxieties, things we can't seem to release—anything that is the opposite of the feeling of well being, or connection to the Essence. It's the pile of bricks in a field of bliss.

In order to discard the energy, it first has to be acknowledged and released. It needs to see the light of day in order to be transformed. Many people fear releasing this energy because they are convinced it's going to hurt more than it's worth. In fact, the opposite is true.

When you face it head on, you're a lot more confident and can more easily deal with whatever you find buried there. I've *never* had it hurt more than I can handle. In fact many times, it wasn't at all painful to resolve. Many times it's a "Eureka!" feeling.

For example, you are hit with a memory of something that happened when you were a child. You were accused of something you didn't do. As a result you weren't allowed to

142

watch Bewitched that night. You haven't thought of it in years, but now you remember it and are then hit with, "Oh, that's why I get so angry when I sense injustice, yet won't let the kids watch TV because I resent that they get what I couldn't have." Many times it really is that trivial and painless! I don't mean to belittle the experience when I say trivial, because it's obviously a very important moment if it can still affect your behavior as an adult. When I say trivial I mean that the fear of facing that cause was a hundred fold greater than the actual moment itself.

By facing these fears and dealing with them, and changing our behavior and reactions to them, walls literally begin to tumble. Whole aspects of your life begin to change for the better because you resonate with "better." As a result, every facet of your life improves because your vibration becomes one of a healthier and happier you.

Ask your body for answers

If you could remember what it felt like to be in your perfect, healthiest shape, you would literally be there right now. Read that sentence again, because it's one of those deceptively simple statements.

It's because you can't remember what it felt like that you can't place yourself there. But there is a simple trick at your disposal: your body knows what its perfect shape is. Ask it to remind you, to bring it about. But then you have to help it along. You have to listen to its clues. If it's telling you not to eat that junk food with all its chemicals and additives and other things that it's loaded with, then listen. Not because the food is fattening, but because your body is telling you that it doesn't remember that being a part of your perfect shape.

Listen to your body when it tells you to move it around in some form of exercise. It's trying to remind you what it feels like to be physical, and that's literally what it means to be in your perfect shape. Your perfect shape is a *physical* manifestation, isn't it? Therefore you must *be* physical. Listen to it with both ears in order to hear what it's telling you about what it takes to feel orgasmically good all the time.

Pay attention to this: If you ask for the answers and then ignore them, your answers might seem to stop coming. And then you might just end up with an illness that "forces" you to listen.

Want an example? Let's say you have a couple of glasses of wine every night. You don't get drunk, in fact most nights you drink so little and so slowly that you really don't catch much of a buzz. It doesn't seem like all that big a deal. But when you start listening to your body, it tells you to back off the wine. No problem, you think, because you don't *need* it, you just enjoy it.

When that evening rolls around, about the time that you would normally uncork the bottle, you're reminded of your body's request. You have a choice. Do you listen to your body, or do you ignore it and reach for the wine? After all, it's only a glass or two. It's not doing any harm.

Well, perhaps it's not doing any major harm. You probably won't get cirrhosis or have any other medical indications. But if your body is telling you to stop, then the wine is lowering your vibe. It's keeping you from being in your perfect form. In addition, you're ignoring what your body is directly telling you, after you *asked* for it to tell you what it needs!

Now, look at it from another angle, but with no guilt— just matter of fact questions. Why did you ignore the clear, plain message you were given? Why did you go ahead and pour a glass of wine? Is it because you have nothing else to do? Is it because it helps to fuzz the harsh lines of reality, to take the sharp edges off the day? Is it because skipping this evening's beverage service isn't going to cause any immediate, instant-gratification type changes in your life so you might as well?

Does the wine help you to feel closer to Spirit? Does it ease the pain you feel when you can't sense the closeness? Has it become a habit that you've denied has a hold on you?

Now try reading that section again, replacing the word "wine" for whatever it is you can't say "no" to. Do you think you can listen to your body now? Has this helped you to see it differently?

Being Soul Connected and Heart Centered

All of these exercises are leading up to your feeling soul connected. This is what religion is *supposed* to teach you to do. Somewhere along the line the message got lost and many people don't know that this is their goal—*this* is their connection to God. They've been taught that the *minister* is the one who knows God and that they can only touch God through him (I'd say "or her" but we all know better. The religions that allow women equal speech don't have as skewed a version of God as the ones who don't.). When I am able to feel the bliss that was outside of the brick wall, I am soul connected. When you are envisioning your healthy, happy you, you are soul connected. It's what we live for. It's why we're here—to learn to be soul connected in spite of adversity or difficult times. We learn lessons from the adversity in order to help us remove obstacles between that connection and us.

> When you're heart centered, you are the authentic *you*— the you that cares enough about yourself to do the right thing for your health and well being.

A helpful tool in becoming soul connected is to heart center. As discussed previously, the heart chakra at the center of your chest is the meeting point for your spiritual, mental and physical energies. It's the melting pot. When you are heart centered, you are able to see with more clarity what's really going on in your life and are able to make better decisions about what's best for you.

When you're heart centered, you are the authentic *you*— the you that cares enough about yourself to do the right thing

145

for your health and well being. *It's the you that cares as much about yourself as you do about others.* So when you're feeling less than 100%, go ahead and heart center. It brings you back to . . . well . . . center!

Here's how, and remember that it really is very easy, probably easier than you expect so you may think you're doing it wrong. We've been trained to believe that everything must be hard or it's not worth doing. Just the opposite is true. Our intent is all it takes. If I intend to be heart centered, then I am. I address the Essence and it gives what I ask for. That's a bit of a leap of faith for many people so here's an exercise that will help you ease into that feeling.

Heart centering helps your thoughts slow down and to open into the energy and power of love. If you're new to this kind of work, try to find a quiet place to release and relax. Once you know how, you can do it anywhere. After you learn how to do it, it sometimes helps to close your eyes when you're centering. But while you're learning, go ahead and just do it as you read along here.

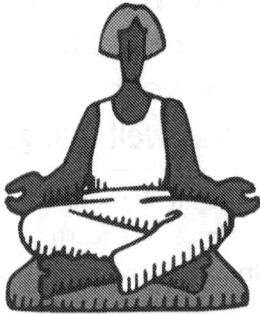

Take a deep breath, in through your nose and out through your mouth. Focus on your breathing being slow, deep and even.

Allow yourself to relax. Bring all your attention to **now**. If you can't focus because the kids are fighting or you're afraid the phone will ring, or you are angry about something, then take care of these things. Take the phone off the hook; tell the kids you need a few minutes of quiet, release the anger and promise to pick it up later if you still feel the need. Call back all the parts of yourself that are scattered. You left some of your energy at work, at the store where you forgot the cat food, in the car that needs cleaning, in your family's fields (They do hold your energy until you bring it back to you. You have some of theirs too. Send it back.) I picture it as wisps of ghosts of myself floating in the scene that holds it. When I

146

call it back, it gets sucked back into my field and integrates itself instantly.

After half a dozen slow breaths focus your attention on the center of your chest, the heart chakra. I imagine that it looks like a swimming pool with an emerald green light filter. Don't worry about seeing it in your mind's eye if this doesn't come easily to you. Just know that it's there. Remember, your intent is all that matters. If you can't "see" it doesn't mean you're doing it wrong, it just means that you don't use that type of visualization. You're still doing it right though.

Imagine the green light expanding, across your chest and filling every area of your body. My visualization for this is as though my body is a gel-like balloon full of green-lit water. This works for me. Find what works for you.

Think of this light as the color of peace, growth and balance. Just rest in this moment as long as you desire. When you feel your outer awareness pulling you back, ask the feeling of peace to remain with you so you can take it with you no matter what you're doing.

Once you're familiar with the process, you'll be able to do it even when stuck in traffic. And I promise, it will make the trip much more pleasant.

Journaling

By keeping a journal, you can keep track of your thoughts and feelings, and just pour your heart out onto the page. You may be surprised at the words that come out, if you just let it go. Free association is another method that you can use in your journal, where you ask a question, write it out at the top of the page, and just fill the page with whatever words come to your mind, even if they seem bizarre and out of place. Pay attention to those words and try to figure out where they came from.

For those people who are more into the computer, you can journal there as well. For me, the computer works better because my hand can't keep up with my brain when I'm trying to write longhand and I can never read my own writing later. At least on the keyboard I stand a chance of getting it all down as it comes. Sit at the keyboard with a blank document open, and type a question. Then close your eyes and let your fingers fly, typing out anything that comes to mind, again, even if it seems bizarre. It may take a while for something to come, because you're drawing a blank or you think that what you're "hearing" is just stuff that you've made up. Go ahead and type it out. As your fingers begin moving, the real stuff will start pouring through.

If nothing comes, try a different way of wording the question. What you write doesn't have to make sense. You can go back later and see if there are any worthwhile needles in the haystack. Some of it will probably be useless, but you will undoubtedly find a gem or two each time you try this.

After a while you'll start to notice trends and patterns that you play out every day, things you were probably unaware of. And, since the journal is a form of Essence, the more you use it the more useful it becomes, just like focusing on the bliss through the brick wall. The more you open up to writing, the more thoughts to write will come. This brings new understanding to issues you're working through and other issues you didn't even know you had!

I hope you're starting to get a feel for how shape shifting affects every aspect of life and that what you focus on grows and becomes stronger. Because once you understand that, it's a real simple leap into the realm of . . .

Magic

As I mentioned earlier, one of the best things I took away from my study of Goddess-based religions is the concept of magic. When you boil it down, it becomes basic metaphysics, and many of the suggestions I've made already are a form of magic. In this section I'll explain a little about how it works and how you can use it in your quest for a healthier body.

By the way, before we go any further, it's worth mentioning that the common fallacy that this is Satanic worship or evil in some way is a **major** misconception. The vast majority of practitioners of this craft don't even believe there is a Satan. They are using the god-force, love energy or Universal Intelligence—they are shape shifting.

How magic works

Kids believe in magic because it makes sense—magic pills and wands and amulets and spells. Of course they work! There is no asking why. They just do. This magic stone has this certain power and that magic spell has a different power. Duh!

If that's the case, then why can't I just blink like Jeannie on *I Dream of Jeannie* or twitch my nose like Samantha on *Bewitched* and make the fat go away? Because Jeannie and Samantha have a TRUE understanding that it works. They simply assume that what they do will work. In fact, they're panicked when it doesn't! They hear a weird, hollow "boing" sound and nothing happens. Then they look around to find out what's interfering with their magic. Usually it's their evil twin cousin plotting to take their man.[87]

The amount of intent, focus and concentration behind those thoughts are what determines whether or not we'll see results.

I know, these are just sitcoms and not real life, and the magic they do isn't the way real magic works. You can't just blink your son-in-law into oblivion. However, you can absolutely create magical changes in your life. But the question remains—when did we stop believing this stuff? That's why it doesn't work for us—we've lost our faith!

Once again, thoughts have substance—electrical impulses sent out to maneuver and manipulate the energies surrounding us *whether we're conscious of it or not*. The amount of

---

[87] Although why anyone would want to steal Darren Stevens is beyond me. He insisted that Samantha deny who she really is!

intent, focus and concentration behind those thoughts are what determines whether or not we'll see results. If we send conflicting thoughts, like, "I am thin and beautiful," one minute but then follow it up with, "Yeah, right," then there isn't a whole lot of focus or intent. You'll get nowhere that way. You've just nullified your initial statement. This is why building a solid intent and focusing on it with all of your concentration is so very important.

The craft of magic, sometimes spelled "magick" to separate it from stage magician's craft, is very powerful. The use of spells to create your reality or your desires *does work*. However, you don't have to be a "witch" to do it. Actually, you don't even have to use spells specifically, but for those who have not yet honed their abilities to manipulate energy otherwise, they are very useful. Heck, you don't even have to call it a "spell" if you're uncomfortable with the word. Just know that the basic concept still boils down to metaphysics.

This is nothing that you haven't already done a million times before—you just didn't do it consciously and/or specifically. Any time that you strongly wished for, prayed for, hoped for, *worked toward* a certain outcome and really focused on getting that result, you were, in essence, spell casting. This is just a creative way of keeping your mind focused—period—end of story. Nothing evil about it. It's a science of faith, not religion—it's metaphysics.

"Evil" only enters the arena if *you* bring it into the mix. Some folks seem to find the concept attractive. But evil doesn't play unless it's invited. Remember, the Essence has no emotions and doesn't distinguish good from evil. Ya gets what ya asks for.

Free will plays an extremely important part here too. When you start messing about with other people, then you are infringing on their free will. I was going to write something about us having no right to do so, but that's incorrect. We have every "right" to do so, if you want to look at it that way. However, it's not so smart. Just because you *can* do something doesn't mean that it's wise. Karma comes into play and you get back what you gave out.

If you work to manipulate someone else, then you too are caught in that web. You can't be heart centered or soul connected when caught in a mess like that. So even though you may have made someone do something against their will, and got what *you* wanted as a result, you're not living your higher truth by doing so. You're also taking advantage of someone else's weakness, which will give you a major karmic kick in the ass. In the end, *nobody* comes out ahead. Instead, work toward the outcome you want in a way that helps everyone involved to become soul connected as a result.

One more thing, before we get into the meat of the topic: please feel free to adapt and change what I suggest here to fit your individual style. I remember when I first started on the spiritual path, I read books on creative visualization and listened to meditation tapes and stuff like that. They would invariably say something like, "Picture yourself in a beautiful place, where you feel totally at ease and relaxed." So I'd see myself on the beach. Then they'd say, "Notice the flowers and trees and find a path into the woods. Follow that path. . ." My reaction was, "Huh??? There are no trees or flowers here! I'm on the friggin' beach!" So I assumed I was just doing it wrong and tried to force my thoughts into what *they* thought was the perfect place. Little wonder it took me a very long time to figure out how to do it right, *for myself.*

So how do we create our reality, a new life for ourselves? What are the components that go into that recipe? Since we're dealing with energy, it can't just be a solid ingredient. So it has to be energetic concepts. The first step in creating a spell is to specify your intent. You must be specific, but not too specific, because otherwise you may limit the results you get. Just remember—you must be careful what you wish for. You just may get it. I know I keep repeating this, but it's essential that you understand this.

Casting a spell

The key to an effective spell is *spelling out* what you want and addressing the Essence with it. First you acknowledge that god-force, and that it is the force with which you'll be working. Then remember that you are in connection with that power and that therefore what you *will*, will be. Name your specific goal and state that this is what you desire, what you will have, for your highest good. For example:

> *(Essence, god force, Universal Intelligence . . . use your favorite word) is within me and all around me. I am a perfect manifestation of (your favorite word). Therefore I call upon its power to make these changes in my body.*
>
> *I use this power to shift my body into a shape that is healthier, more attractive and which is a manifestation of my love of self. I have this power within my abilities and will it to be so, according to my highest good.*
>
> *So mote it be.*[88]

The last line is a traditional way to end a spell, but you can change it to whatever seals the deal for you. It is the same as "amen" at the end of a prayer, so if that works for you, change it to amen. You can even say "make it so," à la Jean Luc Picard, if that strikes your fancy. If you'd rather write it as a poem, go ahead. If you find that what I wrote is too wordy, then change it. Write it in *whatever way works for you.* Just follow the formula.

Once you've found the words for what you want, then you can actually set about putting it into action. Again, there are many ways to do this. You can find some really cool parchment paper and write it out using ink and a quill. Type it onto your computer and print it out with a fancy font. Write

---

[88] This method is adapted from Marion Weinstein's wonderful book *Positive Magic.*

it on a chalkboard in block letters. Whatever makes the message really solid for you is the right way.

If you really want to give it extra oomph, then do a little research. Find out what colors will work best for your specific goal. Check into aromatherapy and find some scent that will trigger your desired results. Use crystals that correspond to your needs. See if there is a god or goddess in mythology who represents the archetype of what you are working toward. Keep the archetype in mind while you work. That's what they're for—this is what witches are doing when they invoke the gods—they're addressing the Essence with a pattern that already exists so they don't have to depend so much upon their own work starting from scratch.

Here are a couple of ideas to get you started. You are only limited by your own imagination, so take these ideas and expand on them:

Take a smallish candle and carve your ideal shape into it, keeping your focused intent in mind the whole time. If you use a colored candle, look into what properties that color possesses so you can incorporate any that will be useful to you.

Then, place the candle in a place where you can sit with it and light it. Read your spell aloud, with conviction, as many times as feels right. If it feels right, you can then burn the paper, sending the energies of your words out with the smoke and flames. (Please, don't set your house on fire. Take the obvious precautions.) Let the candle burn itself out (this is why you use a small candle, because it can take forever for a larger candle to burn itself out and, again, we don't want to burn the house down).

Or, instead of burning the paper, roll it up and tie it with a ribbon; bury it in the yard; put it on your mirror; place it in a box—*again*, whatever appeals to your sense of the magic you're creating. If you feel that you want to dissolve fat, then you can use something like a hardened clump of sugar. As you pour liquid over it and it dissolves, invoke that dissolving power. Try to see everything you do as symbolically forming a healthier, thinner body. When you get up from your chair, make it magic. Petition your muscles to do a little more fat crunching than they usually do. The more you use symbolism like this, the more it expands and becomes a way of life. Soon all of your consciousness will be involved in giving yourself a healthier body and it will be sooooooooo much easier.

If you find that your magic isn't working, then use the failure as a tool to find out what went wrong. Ask yourself why it didn't work. You'll probably get the answer right away. The first thought that comes to your head will quite possibly be your answer. In fact, that answer could be as simple as this, "This stuff doesn't work. You're fooling yourself." If that's the thought that stops you, then you're jumping the gun. You're trying to get to Friday from Monday again.

You've already proven to yourself that you can create a fat body. Look at all your other accomplishments. You can make happen what you've wanted to happen. Even the bad things, see how you've played a part in everything that has ever happened in your past. You have created your life. You know you're good at it. Everything you've done up until this moment is proof. That's pretty powerful! So how come *now* you don't believe you can lose weight?

Always state as your clear intent that no harm will come as a result of what you do.

Remember, this is not mystical, spooky stuff. It's just a fact of how things work. Of course it works. It's the only thing that *does* work. It is. Period. Use it and lose it.

It might also not work easily because you still have some fear in your mind about "evil." You can counteract that problem by making sure that you do not invoke any "gods" or manipulative energies. Always state as your clear intent that no harm will come as a result of what you do. If this is your intent, and the Essence creates with what you give it, then you will only come back with results that truly harm none.

154

Here's another test to see why it isn't working. Listen to your thoughts as you're eating alone, something that you "shouldn't be eating." I bet it sounds something like, "I shouldn't be eating this. I know it makes me fat, and I don't want anyone to see me doing this because they'll know I'm not really trying. But I am trying. I just can't stand it anymore. I've tried so hard and it doesn't work. And this really tastes good. Why can't I have the kinds of foods they can have? They don't have to try to lose weight; they can eat anything they want. How dare they give me a hard time because I want to eat the same foods? It's not my fault that I get fat when I eat!"

Sound familiar? Even if you have a different version of this speech, my point remains the same. Remove the emotion from it and re-read those words. They are all words of denial, of discomfort and pain. This is what you honestly think when you don't think you're thinking. These are the words that are creating your life—*they are **making you fat**.* These are the words you need to overcome—they are your brick wall.

Glamours

Glamours are another type of shift shaping magic that is worth looking at, and it's similar to the "dressing for success" concept. The first time I'd ever really understood what glamour is was after reading Orson Scott Card's *Alvin Maker* series (Highly recommended! Card understands how things work!). One of the characters was trying to disguise who she was, so she used a series of "glamours" to change her appearance. She used hexes and amulets—various magical charms that would each work to change the way she looked.

These aren't old wives tales. They really do work. I think Card's book may have exaggerated how well, but I could be wrong. I haven't pushed the envelope hard enough to know for sure, but I'm really working on it.

The advertising media message seems to be that if you buy their product you'll be beautiful like their skin-and-bones model who's had every form of cosmetic surgery available.

That last part is obviously a false message, but what they say is true, *to a degree.* Actually, the use of their product might help you to look *your* best, but it will not make you look like the model. I know, a big chorus of "Duh!"'s are heading my way, but our subconscious believes their message! We have to remind it otherwise.

Sometimes things are so obvious that we don't think about them anymore. For example, makeup can work wonders to change appearance for the good or bad—check out movie makeup—it changes the way you look! It's become such a part of every day life that we don't even think about it as being special. Imagine life without tools to make you look attractive then think about it again: MAKEUP CHANGES THE WAY YOU LOOK! That's pretty impressive, if you ask me. The same applies to jewelry, accessories and clothing, each of which is a promise of beauty as well.

The danger of the media message lies in believing that you have to buy it from *them.* Many, if not most, of these things, can be had in other ways—make it yourself, trade, gifts, etc. If you choose to buy glamorous things, that's great. Just know that it's not the thing itself, or the company that sells it, that has power. You give it any power it may have.

Good or bad, a glamour is a tool to change your appearance and therefore your life. If you dress like a bum, you'll act like one and be treated as one. This doesn't mean that you will be a bum, at least not immediately, but continue with this glamour and your reality will follow that path until it's true or until you change it. If you dress and make up as though you love yourself, then you begin to feel that way and others will begin to treat you that way. Others will sense the change in your energy field and will respond accordingly, usually without even being aware of it.

Basically, you use the power of association to make a glamour work. If red lipstick makes you feel as sexy as can be,[89] but it makes me feel like a bad Joan Crawford impersonator, then that association will work differently on us, won't it? Once you make a mental decision of what you want to feel, find a physical item to hook it onto. If you decide that you want to become more alive, and wearing the color yellow makes you feel vibrant, then use that as your glamour, or your physical hook.

You can once again use archetypes here. If you wish to exude a certain personality, then wear the things a person with that personality would wear. You see this every single day. You can tell a thug, or a rich person, or a thousand other archetypes by what they choose to wear. By dressing in *that* archetypal manner, you become *that*. The further you are from the goal to begin with determines how long it will take, but keep at it and you **will** create a new reality *within the archetype*. You will not become the person you emulate, you become a person *like* that person.

See what I mean about there being nothing mystical about this stuff? What I just wrote is plain, obvious common sense, but it's totally metaphysics in a nutshell. What makes it difficult for fat people is that we're choosing an archetype that we just can't fit into and so aren't finding success. We're in a large, out of shape body but we want to look like Heather Locklear *overnight*.

It's realistic for a kid to shoot for an archetype like a great athlete like Michael Jordan, or any other hero. The kid simply mimics the hero's behavior. That child is just as capable of achieving that goal as anyone else. It's how much effort he/she puts into making it true that will determine how far he/she goes. Even someone with physical challenges can achieve that goal because Michael Jordan is simply the best he can be. That child can grow into an adult who achieves that exact, same goal. However, that child will never look like

---

[89] I was going to enter a disclaimer about men finding some similar thing to compare, but then realized that some of you guys might just have a tube of Revlon Burgundy Wine. ;-)

Michael Jordan. We simply cannot make another person's body our goal. We need to make their success at looking their best our goal to mimic. Trying to look like someone else will never work and this is why we fail to gain health. We are visualizing us being *them*, not us with our top form!

We can begin to be in our best form by always *looking* our best. Sometimes that best is in a rumpled bathrobe, with morning breath. We don't have to look like a magazine at every moment. Haven't you noticed how cute someone you loves looks when they get up in the morning? You can look good then, too. Put on something that makes you feel good. If you have two robes and one's got a coffee stain on it, don't wait for a special occasion to put on the clean robe. Put on some bunny slippers or something that makes you smile. (I've just told you folks a tremendous amount about myself in the mornings.)

Use glamours as tools when you're off track from being soul-connected. When you're soul-connected you look your best. If you find that you're getting sloppy or frumpy, and are unhappy with that look, then you might want to use glamours to get you back on track.

The simplest things can be used as glamours. I recently found a really pretty color of nail polish that I just had to have. I *never* wear nail polish. I can honestly say that I have gone five years without wearing nail polish. But this one was so cool; it's pink chrome—really shiny (I love gaudy sparkly stuff. I wish we could all wear glitter all the time). Wearing it makes me feel like a girl, after spending my entire life denying that I'm female. So the glamour of the nail polish allows me to feel good about being in this female body. It allows me to connect with the teenaged girl that I was, the one who never wore nail polish and thought being a girl was stupid—the one who never wanted to be a girl—and show her that it's actually kind of fun, when it involves sparkly stuff.

After I started wearing the nail polish, and actually taking care of my nails (I had to learn how to do a manicure) I started wearing more colorful clothing, instead of t-shirts and jeans all the time. These small things led me to many other physical changes, all of which make me *much* more attractive, confident and happy with myself. It's not the fact that I look prettier to others that makes me happier, it's that I made my life more colorful and fun. I don't look like a model and I never, ever will. But I look as good as I can at this moment in time. Tomorrow I'll look even better!

Magic in everyday life

Once you've done your initial magical work there are many more little, but very powerful, ways that you can keep boosting your magic. With everything you do, with every action, every breath, you can continue to reinforce your intent. With every drink of water, say to yourself, "With every drop of water that enters my body, I rinse away excess fat and shift my body into the shape I desire." When you take a shower say, as you're soaping up, "With this shower I wash away excess fat and shift my body into the shape I desire." With every step you take you are walking off excess fat. With every breath, you are breathing life into your new form. With every bite of food that your body (not your mouth) craves you are feeding your new body with what it needs. With every action, you are reinforcing what you want to become. By taking these extra little steps, you are solidly and firmly telling your energy body how to be.

> **With every action, you are reinforcing what you want to become.**

If you want to be creative, you can make your own soap that has your intent within. Take a bottle of unscented body wash and add some essential oils that are specifically known to help with weight loss. As you add the oils, make it a ritual. See the oils as your helpers in dispersing excess fat energy. Pay careful attention to what and how much you put in, because some oils can harm your skin. I personally use grapefruit, orange and lime. Fennel is also useful, but smells like licorice, so go easy on it. Please do your research, because what works for me may not work for you. Use your intuition.

Another good way to use oils is with a diffuser, or even just a bowl of water with a few drops in it. This way you will smell these oils and they will serve as a reminder for you to think thin.

If you're into crystals, which I am in a major way, you can use some of the stones that correspond to weight loss. According to Melody's well-known *Love is in the Earth* guide, the following stones can be helpful: augelite, bertrandite, cassiterite (also known as tinstone), chabazite, chlorite, cinnabar, diaspor, duftite, erythrosiderite, gmelinite, hambergite, heulandite, iolite, laubmannite (when used with acupuncture or acupressure), monazite, black plume opal, overite, Picasso stone, green tourmaline (which is also helpful in working through issues with father or masculine forces), and wilkeite. Frankly, I've only heard of about half of these before looking them up to add them here, but I've also never really looked for some of them before. I'm willing to bet that if you decided to find the right stone for you, you'd end up in a store that sells that stone or it would come to you somehow. Funny how things work that way, isn't it?

In addition to what I've mentioned here, you can find your own methods that appeal to your sense of intuition and creativity. They will work best of all, because they are the methods that have the most meaning for you.

How to burn your imprint

Since our topic of focus is weight loss, and/or a more pleasing form for our bodies, we need to start out with that intent. What do you want your body to look like? Be realistic—remember, you will not look like Pamela Anderson when you're done unless you plan on getting a lot of surgery (even *she* didn't look like that without it!). If that's the case, then you need to add surgery into your plan.

Again, imagine how your body could realistically look, and keep in mind that you've probably aged a few years since you

160

were 17. I know I'll never look like that again. (Of course, I could be wrong—who knows if I could really obtain that body again if I believed strongly enough?) I've had two children and I have stretch marks. I've had gall bladder surgery, so I have a huge scar across my abdomen. My body has changed in ways that it's not worth it for me to sweat over. So I focus on being the best-looking Lisa at this age that I can.

If it helps, try to find pictures of people who look like you would like to look (again, keeping in mind that they have to have the same frame and build that you have). In whatever way works for you, develop a *solid image* of what you intend to be.

Once you've managed to find this image upon which to focus, you will set this as your intent. We're going to burn this image onto our etheric template, or aura. Here is how I do it. Again, please feel free to modify this to fit your own way of doing things.

First, I open myself to the Universal Intelligence by consciously letting my ego drop to the sides. I heart center, filling myself with the green light of love-energy. I see myself as I described earlier, with my skin falling away, leaving nothing but the pure energy that my body and aura really are. I see that the energy is the brightest where I am physically solid, just like a fluorescent or neon tube, with the light dispersing and getting more faint as it gets further from the source. I see, within that light, the form that is currently my body. I acknowledge that this form is made of the same Essence that makes up everything that is, All That Is. Now I ask it to form a slimmer shape, shifting it into the shape I set as my original intent. I ask that this form be my new outline, my new imprint and for the energy to reshape itself into that form.

It may also help you to thank the energy for its assistance, and to thank the energy that used to be your form for its help in reshaping what you will be. Until we can truly realize that there is no separation, then it helps to use our dependence on

161

it for our benefit. Once you've seen that this energy is just that, love-energy, it's much easier to not hate your body for being fat. It's just energy, doing what it's told and going where you've been telling it to go.

You'll be happy to know that this exercise gets much easier over time. At first it may be hard for you to think you're doing it right because you don't think you're seeing what you're "supposed" to see. It will still work just as well the first time though. There is no "supposed to." Just let it be and the more you practice the more you'll see it. Again—it's your *intent* that counts.

You might even want to draw a picture of what you envisioned. It certainly doesn't have to be an artwork. It could just be a line drawing of the shape you want, colored in solidly in the center, but with rays of light and dissolving energy on the outside. Whatever way you pictured it looking when you burned that imprint is best. That's just how I see it. Use crayons and color it if you want. Then you'll be able to easily recall the feeling you had when you burned in the imprint and this will act as a reminder of how great it felt to be that size. The stronger this image is in your mind, the faster and easier you'll become that size.

In this way, we can see ourselves for what we truly are, solidified love energy. And as we are indeed that energy, then we can shape our bodies any way we want. And now we choose to shape them differently. We can see our bodies looking their absolute best, keeping in mind our basic shapes—bone structure, height, etc.—and we can burn that image into our energy field. That is what we will become. Our force of will makes it so.

What we've done, in essence, is compressed the outline of our body to a new place. Now the molecules that exist outside of those boundaries will have to disperse and leave our physical bodies. It can't be done overnight because we're actually removing solid mass with our minds. This takes time. However, if you've burned in this new template, you're more able to bounce insults and discouraging thoughts away. You'll hear, "Boy, you're fat," from someone else or even your own mouth when you look in the mirror. But now you're able to honestly say, "Yeah, I was yesterday. Today I'm thinner."

Don't let those messages have more power than you put into your new template. If you just imprint it once, then sort of just let it go and drift back into your everyday mindset, those fat vibes will just start eating away at the new you, like rust on a neglected car. You must not let go of that new image of yourself. When you get discouraged because you didn't lose 20 pounds overnight, you mustn't listen to your ego telling you, "I told you this wouldn't work. Now come on, let's go eat." Because it will say that, I guarantee it. Instant gratification is *not* something you can always expect from this work.

The Secret of the Universe

This might be a good time to insert some very powerful information I picked up from the *Conversations With God* series by Neale Donald Walsch, in the deceptively simple yet intricate statement, "In the absence of what you are not, what you are, is not." Okay, clear your head for a minute, because this is a thinker. And it is some of the most powerful mojo I've ever laid hands on.

You know how every time you go on a diet, or make some other habit-breaking choice, it seems like you're suddenly overwhelmed by temptation? You make the decision, "I'm not going to cheat on my diet," and the next day someone brings cake or donuts to work, or the vending machine has been

> ### In the absence of what you are not, what you are, is not.
> *Neale Donald Walsch*

magically restocked with your favorite brownies. Happens every time, doesn't it? Wanna know why?

In the absence of what you are not, what you are, is not.

This means, in essence, that nothing can exist without a contrasting truth to distinguish it as different. There is no tall without short, no up without down, no strength without weakness. Once you make a declaration about who you are, the Essence co-creates its contrast as an opportunity to demonstrate your new truth, sometimes in a form we perceive as opposition. How are you ever going to know that you have become a person who doesn't cheat on their diet if you don't have a way to demonstrate that truth?

The beauty of this realization is that you can now view that temptation in an entirely different way: you know how it takes forever to see results when you're dieting? Now you can see instant results! If you have decided to resist temptation, the only way to do so is to be tempted by your old favorites. Instead of caving in, and hating yourself for your "lack of willpower," rejoice that there is proof that the Universe has heard your statement of truth about yourself and is giving you the gift of saying, "Yes, you are! You *are* a person who can sit next to cake all day and not really care! Hooray for you!"

Of course, an easier way to getting around this is to not make declarations about what you're resisting, because then you won't get the difficult proofs. If you, instead, declare that the Universe provides you with yummy yet healthy foods, you won't have to jump this specific hurdle.

Play with this magic formula a bit, and see if it doesn't blow your mind and rock your world. I said at the beginning of this section that it is deceptively simple, and I meant it— hopefully you'll see why.

Sex Magic

Now that we've covered the basics of magic, we can move into an even more fun way of working with energy—sex!

Before we go on, we need to deal with the Sexual Heebie Jeebies[90] first. Do you think sex is perverted? Take a look at its definition. It only indirectly mentions sex. Also observe the etymology. The word originally meant "to turn."

---

[90] Grandaddy of the Nocturnal Heebie Jeebies.

per vert (pər-vûrt´) v.[91]

1. To cause to turn away from what is right, proper, or good; corrupt.
2. To bring to a bad or worse condition; debase.
3. To put to a wrong or improper use; misuse..
4. To interpret incorrectly; misconstrue or distort: *an analysis that perverts the meaning of the poem.*

n. (pûr vûrt)

One who practices sexual perversion.
[Middle English perverten, from Old French pervertir, from Latin pervertere : per-, *per-* + vertere, *to turn*; see wer-[2] in Indo-European Roots.]

So, what do you think? Is sex perverted? Indeed it is, if an effort has been made to turn it into something that it's not. It's not dirty, shameful, or a competition to see who's "better" at it—no matter how hard that message gets hammered into your psyche. Unfortunately, many people can't get off unless it's dirty, shameful, etc., because they've bought into the concept that this is what sex is.

The reason I even bring this aspect of sex up is that it is absolutely imperative that you get over it if you're ever going to make this work in the way you say you want to. If you want to shape shift, and do it quickly, then you must get comfortable with your body and its inherent sexuality. No two ways about it.

Sex is the ultimate creative force—it can create an actual life! How powerful is that? So it stands to reason that one can use orgasm to seal in your wish list! Yes, even fat people (although society has tried hard to convince everyone otherwise)!

[91] *The American Heritage® Dictionary of the English Language, Fourth Edition Copyright © 2000 by Houghton Mifflin Company.*

The buildup to sexual climax is similar to the buildup of energy when manifesting or spell casting. Allowing oneself to drop aside the ego and open to the energy of orgasm is what creation is all about. Sure, women can get pregnant without orgasm but that's because feminine is passive and internal. Masculine is aggressive and external. That doesn't mean that you can't have them if you want to though.

While sex is obviously designed for procreation, a lot of people don't realize that it can be used for creation of other things than babies. It's the most powerful creative energy there is, so it only follows that it can be used to create the birth of new things and adventures. Through orgasm, one connects and communicates with the Oneness, with god, love-energy, Universal Intelligence, etc., especially if all the participants are aware of and enjoying each other's pleasure. This is where the true bond comes in.

Similar to basic magic, the buildup of intent and focus are most important. If you intend to use sex magic, you need to set the stage. This is not to say that you can't use an unexpected "quickie" in the same way, but the more effort that is spent on laying out the intent, the more powerful the results. In addition, you don't have to have a partner to do this. In fact, for some people it may be more effective to do it alone because their partner may not be the type of person with whom they can easily do the work. (If you just said "ewww!" to doing it alone, then you need to work on your sexuality issues. Sexual hang-ups are about the biggest manifestation killers of all time.)

Keep yourself soul-connected because this is powerful mojo and what you ask for you will get.

Once again, I'll lay out the caveat that you should *use what works for you*. My method may leave you cold, so keep that in mind when planning what you'll do.

First, since sex is specifically a use of our bodies, we need to learn to appreciate them. Sex is a pretty astonishing thing and we can't do it without them. Well, okay, some people can *think* themselves into orgasm, but they still feel it in their bodies. (A fun trick . . . try it sometime.)

Start out by adorning your body in a way that you find sexual. If that means lingerie, hot oil, nipple clamps,[92] have at it. Just let your body know that sex is in the offing. Use perfumes, makeup, jewelry, whatever. But make sure that what you're doing sets a *positive* stage. If you're into S&M, you may want to set aside the leather for this trip, if part of how you get your kicks is feeling bad about yourself or dominating someone else.[93] We're aiming at loving ourselves, not being punished or punishing others. Keep yourself soul-connected because this is powerful mojo and what you ask for **you will get.** Just because it doesn't happen overnight doesn't mean it's not barreling down in your direction.

Dressing (or undressing) for the part kicks off the energies. You can then set the physical stage in a way that continues to build the energy. Incense, candles, lights turned low, all the stereotypical mood enhancers apply. Add your own, if I've forgotten to mention it. You might smudge the room with some sage, which really helps to clear negative energy. Surround the bed, or wherever, with a curtain of smoke, creating a space within which magic will happen. Perhaps you can picture a bubble of energy forming around the bed (let's just assume it's a bed for brevity's sake). Continue this energy/mood build up until it feels right for you. Keep your thoughts on your goal, which is making magic.

Again, details will be different for everyone, but once the physical sexual buildup has begun, allow your mind to focus

---

[92] Whatever floats your boat—different strokes for different folks. And no, this is NOT a confession of any sort.

[93] Incidentally, you can use your sexual "quirks" to solve your mystery. They are amazing tools to let you know what your creative thoughts are.

on your body now, and how you would like for it to look. Really allow the love/Essence/Universal Intelligence in, loving your body as it is now—remembering that it is only energy that has shifted your shape into a way that *you have asked it to*. If you start to feel self-conscious because of how you look, if self-loathing creeps in, remember that this is your ego, trying to ruin your good time. Tell it to leave.

As you build to orgasm, begin to see yourself as actually looking like your goal body. Feel and act like you actually have that body. *Be* that body, right now! Be as sexual as you would be if you were thinner. See and feel your body changing. See the energy-that-is-you transforming. See your shape *shifting*. Send your physical form the unlimited, infinite love-energy that you are accessing from the god-source All That Is and burn in that imprint. *Do not* be self-conscious. Fight that reaction with the love/Essence within. If it helps, silently chant an affirmation:

Allow your old ideas about yourself to die, and the new one to be created.

"I am love. I am love. I am love." If you want to laugh, laugh. If you want to cry, cry. Whatever fits the moment is the wave upon which you'll ride. When you feel you can't get any higher, go higher. When you feel you can't take any more, take some more. When you know you will die if you let it build more, *let it build more! Allow your old ideas about yourself to die, and the new one to be created.*

At the moment of orgasm, release the image you've burned in to your template to Universal Intelligence to do with what it will. Then rest assured that it will be. The stronger your conviction, the sooner it will happen.

The reason I stress so adamantly that sex magic must be done with a pure, loving heart, is that I'm convinced that the only way we can truly access the ultimate power, the actual Essence of god, is if we are doing it with no ill intent whatsoever, only with pure, raw love.[94] It's the only way we can use its power in its unbridled form. Only when our intent is loving does the key fit the lock—it's the only way we will be let in the door—and only then does Spirit give its full sanction for us to crank up the volume full blast.

To be sure, "impure" magic does have access to some of that power because, as I've said over and over, *energy itself is neutral. It has no feelings, no judgments, no good, no bad. It's waves and empty space. It just is and it is every thing.* But I am absolutely convinced that impure magic cannot access the same wallop-packing power that intent with love can because it's got a filter installed, making it "impure." In addition, what it creates is perverted ... corrupted. What it creates isn't a duplicate of love, it's a duplicate of that filter. What it creates is a malshifted shape.[95]

I'm aware that this process may be difficult for many people. At one time it would have been literally impossible for me, because I grew up with all sorts of twisted ideas about sex and sexuality. You know how I got over them? I explored my sexuality, like I'm recommending you do.

Sex isn't called "making love" for nothing. This is the best way to truly connect to love energy and if that's *the least* that you do, you're still better off than those who don't even try.

---

[94] Which is, after all, the body of god!
[95] On a side note, the argument can be made that if everything is made of Essence/god/love/Universal Intelligence/etc., then so is that filter. Indeed, that's true, so even that malshifted shape is pure love. But it's in the form of the filter you put on it. And if you've decided that this filter has had a part in creating something you don't want or like anymore, then you need to drop that filter!

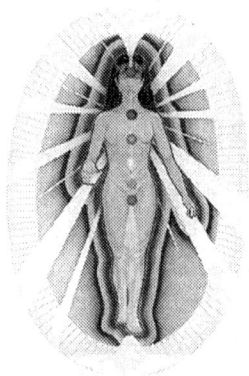

OTHER FUN TOOLS

By now it should be obvious that excess weight is an incredibly complex, multi-dimensional issue, and it may help you to look into some other interesting ways to get to the bottom of your own cause and effect. What caused you to allow the weight gain to begin with? This is not to say that it's "your fault." It is, however, your responsibility. We're not laying blame, remember? It might be easier to see it as a mystery that you're trying to solve, following clues that will lead you to the answers you're seeking. The fact is, you have too much weight on your frame and you want it gone. The following are brief descriptions of some fun tools to help you discover how to do it. See what captures your interest and look into it further.

Acupuncture

I've already told you one of my experiences with acupuncture, but in addition to that one specific amazing incident, acupuncture is useful in removing energy blocks. Those energy blocks can be found to have solidified into fat, disease, tumors, cysts, etc. Remember that our bodies are just densely packed molecules. By removing the blocks, our energy flows more smoothly and will eventually settle into a more healthy form.

Acupuncture, an almost 5,000-year-old practice, is based on the premise of thousands of energy meridians running through your body like electrical wiring. Life force energy, or chi, travels along those meridians. Where these meridians meet are tiny chakras—the acupuncture points—and these points correspond to various organs. The point isn't necessarily where the organ is, however. Women even have a uterus point in their ears.

Their method of diagnosis is different from what we're used to as well. They take a look at how symptoms relate to each other, what your tongue looks like, how you smell, etc., and they measure twelve radial pulses in your wrist. After diagnosing the whole body, not just broken parts like a bad carburetor, the acupuncturist will place tiny needles into the points that will help to reconnect the energy flow needed to help your body to heal.

Hypnotherapy

This is one of my favorites. Talk about exploring the mysteries of the mind! A good hypnotherapist can assist you in unearthing buried causes for all sorts of conditions in your life. You may find that you've completely forgotten something that happened when you were small to cause you to be unable to stop eating unhealthy foods. Maybe it was something as simple as one of your siblings swiping your Halloween candy, so you learned to snarf all the chocolate before anyone else could get it. Maybe you've had some sort of traumatic experience that causes the weight. By uncovering them through hypnotherapy, you should be able to gently and lovingly clear issues from your mind and energy field.

A myth about hypnosis is that you'll be unconscious. Quite the opposite—you'll be in a state similar to deep meditation but totally aware. And no, you won't come out of it barking like a dog, or clucking like a chicken. Stage hypnosis and clinical hypnosis are two entirely different animals (Sorry. Me and puns . . . I can't pass them up.).

Meditation

With this powerful tool, you are able to access literally unlimited amounts of information. In this relaxed state, you can more easily communicate with Universal Intelligence and ask for guidance or the answers you seek.

Much of what has been discussed in this book is a form of meditation. Use meditation tapes in the beginning, if that's helpful. And, at the risk of really beating this point to death, don't worry about doing it wrong. There is no such thing. Your soul-connected intent will *always* lead you in the right direction. And have fun with it! This is better than any toy you'll ever find under the Christmas tree.

Past life regression

In short, past life regression is a method through which you can access information about your other lives and the issues you carry with you into this lifetime. It's similar to a hypnotherapy session except that we are guided to find the root of an issue we're currently working through from another lifetime.

Reincarnation is a staple for many religions and was apparently removed from the Bible when those in power thought their followers might not toe the line if they believed they had more than one chance for redemption.

The concept is that we live many lives, in many circumstances. In this way our souls can experience all that life has to offer. There is no way that we could do it all in one lifetime, so we do it all in many lifetimes. We are the rapist in one and the rape victim in another. We are the murderer and murdered. We are the loved and we are the hated. We carry our experiences with us in our soul's memory and can access them when meditating, under hypnosis, while dreaming, during a regression, and other ways as well.

Whether or not you believe in reincarnation is something you need to decide for yourself. However, if you don't believe in reincarnation, you can look at past life regression as a creative way that your mind is telling you stories that pertain to what you're doing now. Take the symbolism and look at it like a dream that you're interpreting. It doesn't matter if you were really Pocahontas or not. The information is there. What you do with it is up to you.

At one point in my life I had horrendous TMJ problems. Both sides of my jaw clicked and crunched whenever I would chew something and from time to time my whole jaw would get locked into position. If I yawned, my jaw would lock tight but my muscles, needing to yawn, would force it out of that lock and it would make a loud, painful pop. One morning I woke up with a strong pain in my left jaw joint and nothing was making it go away. My doctor had no idea what was wrong (HMO—go figure). So I went to my favorite hypnotherapist. We did a past life regression that I found simply fascinating.

Apparently, at one time I was living as a young boy, early teens, with my current partner as my older brother. I was smarter than he was and a bit of a showoff, and this made him hate me. Somehow I had proven him wrong in front of many other people and he was just livid. He picked up a sledgehammer and smashed me in the left side of my face, tearing my jaw completely off my face, killing me.

Gnarly story, indeed. But how on Earth did that relate to my current pain? Well, my partner and I were arguing over the solution to a problem. I knew I was right but I didn't want to speak up and tell him he was wrong. I didn't want to make him angry with me so I kept my mouth shut. The day after this argument is the morning I woke up with my jaw hurting so badly. The interesting thing is that he isn't even the type of person to get angry when you disagree with him. He would never be violent with me, and I'm not afraid of him. But my subconscious was afraid of angering him because I feared his retribution. (Perhaps he learned something from that past life as well, like being angry to the point of violence causes death and bad karma.)

174

But the pain went away *during* the regression. When I got home, I brought up what I needed to say, and my jaw began hurting, but once I stated my case the pain was gone and never returned. And I'm happy to say he didn't bash me in the mush for saying it.

Again, it really doesn't matter if that really happened in Moscow, 1794. The symbolism was vivid enough for me to be able to solve the problem after its analysis. So don't allow skepticism to keep you from exploring this powerful tool.

Soul retrieval

Soul retrieval is one of the more fascinating things I've tried. Again, like reincarnation, you don't necessarily have to believe in it for it to work. If you're skeptical, then just look at it as symbolic. Having said that, let's proceed without any more disclaimers.

The concept is that as we grow up, traumas or jarring incidents cause us to leave a part of ourselves, our energy, behind. We leave parts of our energy with a person or place, perhaps a place we didn't want to leave or had difficulty leaving. I mentioned this earlier, how when heart centering you need to call your energy back to yourself.

In addition, people with a more powerful presence than us can take ours against our will, for example, an abusive spouse or a psychic vampire. Someone by whom we're intimidated probably owns some of our energy or is very like the one who does. Our inability to stand up for ourselves is an indication that part of us may be missing. All of these pieces and parts need to come back to us before we can be whole. We can call back a lot of it on our own, but if we aren't aware that it's gone, or someone else is holding it, then we may need help. That's where a Shamanic practitioner comes in.

The Shaman makes an energetic "journey" into the ethers where intelligent energy lives outside of the physical realm and gathers pieces of yourself to bring back to you. Once those pieces are returned you integrate them into your current

175

life. For example, if a part was you at 14, and it's been gone for 20 years, it needs to catch up with all the happenings of the last 20 years. After it has stretched into the new form and fits the current you, you will then have access to the abilities and talents that this part took with it.

At this point in this writing, I've had four soul retrievals done and every one has made a massive impact on my life—all for the better.

Reiki

Several years ago I received my first Reiki treatment. At the time I really didn't know what it is, I just knew that it was supposed to be reputable energy work and I'm always interested in trying something new. The woman had me lie on a table, with lights dimmed, incense, plinky music, etc., and she laid her hands over me projecting Reiki energy. That evening, not feeling too much different and kind of disappointed that it wasn't bigger than it was, I was lying in bed, almost asleep. Suddenly I felt my entire spinal column wake up. I could "see" all the vertebrae and the nerves that are connected directly to it, and it was all lit up and energized. It made a buzzing noise that was really very cool and I felt better than I ever had before. It reminded me of my acupuncture experience.

The next day I looked into what Reiki is, and eventually ended up being attuned to the third level, Master/Teacher. An attunement is different from a treatment. With a treatment you receive Reiki. With an attunement you become a channel for Reiki. There are three levels because it's powerful stuff. If done too quickly it can short out your system and cause some messy fallout.

There is a great deal written about Reiki that is much better than I could begin to touch here, but in essence Reiki is healing energy. It is the ultimate Essence. The word itself means Universal Life Force in Japanese and "Reiki" energy, by that name, has been used for healing since the mid 1900's. Reiki isn't new, however. It's the same healing energy used by healers since time began. Reiki is what Christ used—his was more powerful than ours usually is because he was truly soul-connected. He had no doubt it would work. However, many "miracles" have been performed with Reiki by "mere mortals."

This entire book has been about how we are energy beings, and how if we're soul-connected we can create positive, loving changes in our lives. Until we are soul-connected, we either aren't prepared to handle this type of energy or we don't know we have it. A Reiki attunement awakens us to the fact that we have full access. I strongly recommend Reiki attunement for everyone, or at least Reiki treatments.

Attunements are easy to get and can cost anywhere from no charge to thousands of dollars, depending on the teacher's school of thought. Many people believe that Reiki should be shared freely and will *give* attunements. Others believe that the attunements must be paid for in order for there to be an exchange of energy, and charge a sometimes hefty fee. Some people won't believe they got anything if they didn't pay for it, so they don't want a free attunement. So there is something for everyone. If you want it free, you'll find it (an internet search for "free Reiki attunement" will show you what a growing community it is). If you think you get what you pay for, find a Reiki teacher to pay. Both scenarios are reasonable and are both perfect exchanges of energy.

Dreams

Dream interpretation—what fun! It's like being given a foreign film without dubbing or subtitles and being told to figure out what the storyline is! You can only use the symbolism you see in actions, colors, body language, characters and apparent plot line to figure it out. A good director uses symbolism everywhere in a movie so if you don't follow the dialog you can still get the gist.

The trick to dream interpretation is to not take the storyline or characters too literally. People in your dreams aren't usually really them, they represent an aspect of yourself—they are an archetype symbol. The fact that we're close to them makes it difficult to see this and to remove them from the analysis. We try to insert them into the storyline, "I dreamed my husband cheated on me, but he wouldn't do that, would he?" We begin to doubt loved ones because of a dream we had.

The dream is probably trying to tell you that a part of yourself isn't being very faithful or loyal to you. The fact that it's represented by someone who's supposed to care for you means that it's the part of yourself that should be doing this job. This archetype, within yourself, is being disloyal to your quest for soul-connection.

Unfortunately, I'm not enough of an expert to truly advise on dream interpretation, but can certainly recommend reading the works of Carl Jung. If that's too heavy for you, there are many great books written about his work that are much easier to understand.

Ask for help

You can ask for strength. Project onto Universal Intelligence your request for help if you feel you can't do it alone. Ask to be reminded throughout your day what you're trying to do and for the strength of will to not fall backwards into old ways of thinking. The Essence will give you what you ask for, because your thoughts are things, remember?

You have to *ask* for help or you won't get it easily. If you don't ask for help, it will either not come at all, or it will come in a hard way.

Your subconscious knows where it's steering you and it will put you there no matter how hard you try to impede it. When you interfere with your higher truth, life gets hard and puts you in situations to *force* you in the right direction.

If you really need the help and still don't ask, the subconscious will give it to you in the form of "nudges" and it doesn't care how difficult the nudge is. The harder the nudge, the harder the subconscious is trying to get you to shake yourself out of your fog and pay attention. "Get back on track," is what it's screaming.

By not asking for help from Spirit, you're inviting interference from family and friends, people not minding their own business and messing with your world to force you to take action. You're asking for accidents, illnesses, arrests, excess fat, broken hearts, homelessness and audits.

When you ask for help, your subconscious puts you in the right place at the right time, meeting the right people, letting money fall into place and helps you to attain glowing health. You are, in a sense, rewarded for *asking* for help by *receiving* it!

Help feels fantastic! It's like getting an extra scoop of ice cream. It's like a birthday party when you're a kid and getting all the presents you asked for. It's having that model airplane fall together and look like an expert did it. It's Fruit Stripe gum.

Sometimes that help will look more like a "test," if we don't pay attention. If, the day after you ask for strength, you see a size 5 woman eating an ice cream cone, don't just automatically think, "That skinny bitch," and "Ice cream makes *me* fat." Instead, see it as a reminder that, "She doesn't think this will make her fat, why should I?" Your help may just be a little tickle, a little nudge, to put you back on track. The more help you need, the stronger the message, so watch for it. If you don't see the answer, you'll keep getting nudged until you do.

Once we ask for help, then we can concentrate on going back to loving our body, because we're working with it, not fighting against it and hating it. We know that help is coming so we can relax and let it come.

What To Do When You're Stuck

It is inevitable that, from time to time, you will be stuck at the same weight for a while. It's at this point that many of us give up trying. It's easy to stick to something when you're seeing results, but when you're doing everything you've been doing and you're not losing any more weight, most of us quit trying and go back to old habits.

Usually we're told that we've hit a "plateau" and that we need to cut down on the calories/carbs even more. Has this ever worked for you? My response is typically, "I'm not cutting back another single calorie/carb. I'm starving as it is."

If you're doing everything "right," it's been working well and all of a sudden you stop, then this is a sign that you've finished working through the previous issue. It's time to move on to the next one. You can either skate on that same level for a while, lapse into old habits, or you can jump right on the issue that causes you to lapse into old habits!

This is what stops us—falling back into unhealthy patterns. If we could just stick with the good vibes and expand upon them, then our lives would be so much different! We'd be healthy and happy and wealthy and wise, and birds would sing. But for some reason we just keep falling back.

It's a lack of soul-connection.

Make every action a concerted effort to either stay on track or get back on track. If you blew it, blow it off. Become obsessed with being *healthy*, not with being thin. Get back on and keep going. Begin centering again and concentrate on those flashes of pure Essence, those healthy, happy you vibes that you created. Focus on them and they will continue to grow again, right where you left off. Keep it up. Surf the Essence.

Break down the brick wall by focusing on the bliss. Soon you'll realize that it's been reduced to rubble that you can step right over and leave behind. When you're on the outside, you'll look back and see that this seemingly insurmountable wall was simply made of *fat*.

You're already shape shifting. But now, you're doing it *consciously*.

CONCLUSION

I hope that you've come to the end of this book with a sense that you really *can* do something to shift the shape of your life for the better, whether or not losing weight is part of that change. You may find, after all this reading, that you like your body just the way it is. If that's the case, fantastic!

You can use the techniques I've outlined for making other changes, too. For although the subject of this book was weight loss, the core methods work for anything you want to transform. I didn't invent these metaphysical processes—they're Universal Laws. I simply applied them to one specific subject that has been somewhat neglected in this field. You can do the same.

We create our lives—good, bad or indifferent. *You* choose which energetic waves you're going to surf. You might as well ride the happy, healthy ones!

Namaste,
Lisa

About the author

Lisa Bonnice has been studying metaphysics and the magical arts for over 20 years, including pursuing a degree in metaphysics.

She has earned her living as a stand-up comedienne, humor columnist, television reporter, writer for *Hollywood Revue*—a television variety show, editor for Future Medicine Publishers' *Alternative Medicine—The Definitive Guide* and spent over five years as a multi award-winning affiliate writer and producer for MSNBC.com.

Lisa has also had the honor of addressing the Spiritual Caucus at the UN, while serving in her role as Southern Regional Coordinator for Humanity's Team.

Her original book, *Addressing the Goo—the metaphysics of weight loss*, caught the attention of Neale Donald Walsch, best-selling author of the *Conversations With God* series. Walsch loved the book but hated the title. He suggested that Lisa change the title, but that would mean reconceptualizing and rewriting the entire book.

As Lisa's momma didn't raise no fools, she took the advice of that expert in the field. She retitled and rewrote the original book. You hold the result in your hand.

Lisa has two daughters—Kristina and Stacy—who turned out to be very cool people and are terrific fun to be around, and three really fun little Indigo grandkids. She and Jeff currently reside in Florida.

Oh yeah—she's also lived a zillion or so times.